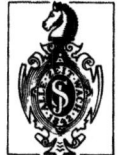

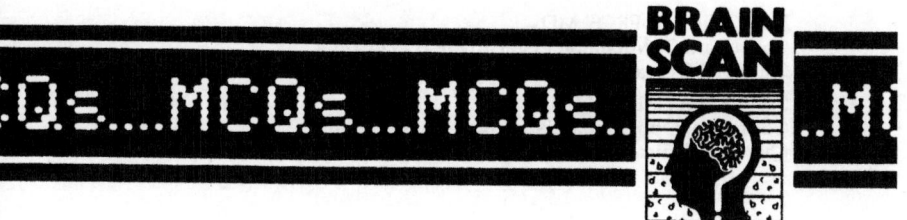

N.R. Galloway · S.A. Vernon

Ophthalmology

Springer-Verlag
London Berlin Heidelberg New York
Paris Tokyo

N.R. Galloway, FRCS, MD
Consultant Ophthalmologist, University Hospital,
Queen's Medical Centre, Nottingham NG7 2UH, UK

S.A. Vernon, MB, FRCS, DO
Consultant Opthalmologist, University Hospital,
Queen's Medical Centre, Nottingham NG7 2UH, UK

Publishers note: the 'Brainscan' logo is reproduced by courtesy of The
Editor, *Geriatric Medicine*, Modern Medicine GB Ltd

ISBN-13:978-3-540-19516-0   e-ISBN-13:978-1-4471-1624-0
DOI: 10.1007/978-1-4471-1624-0

British Library Cataloguing in Publication Data
Galloway, N.R. (Nicholas R)
Ophthalmology
1. Man. Eyes. Diseases
I. Title II. Vernon, S.A. (Stephen Andrew) 1955–   . III. Series 617.7
ISBN-13:978-3-540-19516-0

Library of Congress Cataloging-in-Publication Data
Galloway, N. R.
Opthalmology. (Brainscan MCQ's) Questions based on: Common eye
diseases and their management/N.R. Galloway. 1985.
1. Eye—Diseases and defects—Examinations, questions, etc. I. Vernon, S.
A. (Stephen Andrew), 1955–   . II. Galloway, N. R. Common eye diseases
and their management. III. Title. IV. Series. [DNLM: 1. Eye diseases—
examination questions. WW 18 G174o] RE46.G34 1985
Suppl. 617.7'0076 88-6437
ISBN-13:978-3-540-19516-0

Phototypesetting by Goodfellow & Egan, French's Mill,
French's Road, Cambridge.

2128/3830-543210

Preface

This series of multiple choice questions is based on the textbook *Common Eye Diseases And Their Management* (1985), also from Springer-Verlag. The questions have been grouped to fit in with the chapter headings in the latter. Many of the questions are supported by expanded answers but further information should be sought in the textbook. The format of the questions has been arranged so that the number of true or false answers varies and we have taken pains to eliminate the ambiguities which tend to creep into multiple choice question papers.

In compiling these questions, we have attempted to incorporate a number of key facts and it will be seen that these have occasionally been repeated for emphasis. A surprisingly large amount of information is contained in questions and answers, and simply reading through both can be a useful learning experience in itself.

The questions have been aimed at the medical student level but it is hoped that they may be of some value to general practitioners outside ophthalmology and perhaps also to postgraduates.

The computerised Kuder–Richardson reliability index, which measures the consistency of a student's performance, has shown these questions to be reliable in assessing a students' knowledge. A sample of these questions has been tested in another medical school and we understand that students' marks there equate well with the results from essay questions.

In our university, the medical students achieved a mean of 49.6% with a standard deviation of 12.1%, a negative marking system similar to those used for postgraduate examinations was used.

Reading through MCQs is becoming a popular method of learning, considering the numerous similar publications which are available in other subjects. We feel that a student will benefit from the extra knowledge obtained in this way provided that the answers are not used before thought has been given to the question. Critics of MCQs claim that an "unfair advantage" may be gained by reading through questions prior to the exam. Even if this is so, questions can be carefully altered for examination purposes, if this is thought to be necessary, to discourage "parrot fashion" learning. In view of the number of questions available in this publication, we doubt that this will be necessary.

Nottingham   N.R. Galloway
November 1987   S.A. Vernon

Contents

1. *Introducing the Eye*

Questions

Q.1.1   **The structure of the cornea:**

    a. The corneal epithelium merges with the sclera
    b. The epithelium on the anterior surface of the cornea is continuous with the conjunctival epithelium
    c. The corneal epithelium is a single layer of cells
    d. The corneal epithelium contains keratin
    e. The corneal endothelium is not capable of replication.

Q.1.2   **Surface anatomy of the globe:**

    a. The opening of the tarsal glands lies exterior to the lash roots
    b. The fleshy lump at the inner canthus is called the lacrimal carbuncle
    c. The upper and lower lacrimal puncta both drain tears to the lacrimal sac via the canaliculi
    d. The junction of cornea and conjunctiva is called the limbus
    e. Free drainage of tears helps to maintain normal intra-ocular pressure

Q.1.3   **Orbital nerves and muscles:**

    a. Pupillomotor fibres run in the IIIrd cranial nerve
    b. The lateral rectus muscle is supplied by the IVth cranial nerve
    c. The IVth cranial nerve passes through the optic foramen
    d. Corneal sensation is mediated through the ophthalmic division of the Vth cranial nerve
    e. The inferior oblique muscle arises from the anterior part of the floor of the orbit

Q.1.4   **Vascular supply:**

    a. The ophthalmic artery is a branch of the external carotid
    b. The vortex veins drain the choroid
    c. The fovea is avascular
    d. The lacrimal artery is a branch of the internal carotid
    e. The central retinal artery lies within the optic nerve during part of its course

For answers see over

Answers

A.1.1 a. F—It merges with the conjunctival epithelium.
b. T
c. F—The corneal epithelium usually consists of six layers of cells.
d. F—The corneal epithelium is non-keratinised stratified squamous in type.
e. T—This is generally accepted but replication may occur in exceptional circumstances.

A.1.2 a. F
b. F
c. T
d. T
e. F

A.1.3 a. T
b. F
c. F
d. T
e. T

A.1.4 a. F
b. T
c. T
d. F
e. T

Q.1.5   The uvea:

   a. The uvea is not pigmented
   b. Iridocyclitis means recurrent inflammation of the iris
   c. Iridocyclitis is the same as anterior uveitis
   d. The iris is all derived from mesoderm
   e. The dilator muscle of the iris is sympathetically innervated

Q.1.6   Arterial supply:

   a. The anterior ciliary arteries are from muscular branches of the ophthalmic artery
   b. The posterior ciliary arteries are branches of the anterior ciliary artery
   c. The central retinal artery has no equivalent vein
   d. The vortex arteries supply the choroid
   e. The central retinal artery is an "end artery"

Q.1.7   Innervation of the globe:

   a. There are no pain fibres within the eye
   b. The sympathetic fibres in the long ciliary nerve mediate constriction of the pupil
   c. The parasympathetic supply in short ciliary nerves produces meiosis
   d. Nerve fibres run in the inner part of the retina
   e. The conjunctiva is less sensitive to light touch than the cornea

Q.1.8   The lens:

   a. Is fully grown at the age of 25 years
   b. Moves backwards in accommodation
   c. Forms from surface ectoderm
   d. Is firmly adherent to the vitreous in the elderly
   e. Is usually dislocated in Marfan's syndrome

For answers see over

Answers

A.1.5
  a. F—The uvea consists of the choroid, ciliary body and iris. All three areas contain pigmented cells.
  b. F—Iridocyclitis means inflammation of the iris and ciliary body.
  c. T
  d. F—The posterior pigment layer and dilator muscle are derived from neural ectoderm.
  e. T—Fright results in a dilated pupil.

A.1.6
  a. T—These arteries can be seen running forward from the rectus muscles during squint surgery.
  b. F—The posterior ciliary arteries are direct branches of the ophthalmic artery within the muscle cone.
  c. F
  d. F—The vortex veins drain the choroid.
  e. T—As witnessed in the clinical picture during central retinal artery occlusion.

A.1.7
  a. F—Pain fibres are found throughout the uvea, particularly so in the iris.
  b. F—Dilatation not constriction.
  c. T
  d. T—The major retinal vessels are partially embedded in this layer.
  e. T—Ingrowing lashes may only be perceived when they touch the cornea.

A.1.8
  a. F—Growth continues slowly throughout life.
  b. F—it moves forwards.
  c. T
  d. F—Otherwise intracapsular extraction would inevitably lead to vitreous loss.
  e. T—Partial dislocation is a feature of the syndrome.

Questions

Q.1.9 The ciliary body:

a. Produces aqueous by ultrafiltration alone
b. Has a muscular element that can be paralysed by atropine
c. Is a highly vascular structure
d. Stops producing aqueous at intraocular pressures above 35 mm Hg (4665 Pa)
e. Is innervated by parasympathetic fibres which travel with the oculomotor nerve

Q.1.10 The vitreous:

a. Contains no collagen
b. Contains hyaluronic acid
c. Is not firmly attached to the retina
d. Is more fluid in myopes
e. Is a poor growth medium

Q.1.11 The lacrimal gland:

a. Is an endocrine gland
b. Is parasympathetically innervated
c. Produces basal tear secretion
d. Lies in the lower outer quadrant of the orbit
e. Is involved in Sjögren's syndrome

For answers see over

Answers

A.1.9 a. F—Ultrafiltration and secretion play a role.
b. T
c. T—It is part of the uvea, the vascular coat of the eye
d. F—Much higher pressures are required before ischaemia causes cessation of aqueous production.
e. T

A.1.10 a. F
b. T
c. F—It is attached at the ora serrata, around the optic disc and along the retinal vessels.
d. T
e. F—Pathogenic microorganisms can destroy the eye in 48 hours if introduced into the vitreous.

A.1.11 a. F—It is an exocrine gland.
b. T
c. F—It produces reflex tear secretion.
d. F—The upper outer quadrant.
e. T—Rheumatoid arthritis and inadequate tear secretion.

2. *Primary Eye Care Problems*

Long Sight, Short Sight

Q.2.1 Spectacles
a. Myopic glasses make the eyes look smaller
b. Hypermetropia increases in middle age
c. Short sight is the same as hypermetropia
d. Acute narrow angle glaucoma is more common in short-sighted patients
e. Contact lenses give better distance acuity than glasses in a high myope

Q.2.2 Testing vision:
a. A patient should be asked to view the Snellen test type through a pinhole if glasses have been left at home
b. Indirect ophthalmoscopy allows a binocular, wide field view of the fundus
c. The gonioscope is used for viewing the conjunctival fornix
d. The optic disc cannot be seen with the slit lamp
e. A perimeter is used to measure the corneal circumference

Q.2.3 More facts about visual testing: true or false:
a. The Maddox rod is found in the retina
b. A synoptophore is a unit of eye pigmentation
c. 8% of men fail the Ishihara test
d. The eye is too large in axial myopia
e. The converging power of the lens is usually too great in index myopia

Q.2.4 The axial length of the eye may be measured by:
a. Keratometry
b. Exophthalmometry
c. Ophthalmoscopy
d. 'a' scan ultrasound
e. Calipers

For answers see over

Answers

A.2.1 a. T—And the line of the cheek shifts inwards when seen through the spectacles.

b. F—Apparent increase in hypermetropia is due to progressive weakness of accommodation.

c. F—Short sight is the same as myopia.

d. F—Acute narrow angle glaucoma is more common in hypermetropes.

e. T—In myopia the image size is increased when the correcting lens is brought nearer the eye.

A.2.2 a. T—The pinhole eliminates the effect of refractive error.

b. T—It is especially useful for the examination of patients with suspected retinal detachment.

c. F—It is used to examine the angle of the anterior chamber.

d. F—By incorporating a special lens in front of the patient's eye, it is possible to examine the fundus with the slit lamp.

e. F—It is used to examine the visual field.

A.2.3 a. F—It is an optical device which converts a point source of light into a line and is used for measuring the angle of a squint.

b. F—It is an instrument for assessing binocular function.

c. T

d. T

e. T

A.2.4 a. F—This measures the radius of curvature of the cornea.

b. F—This measures relative forward or backward displacement of the globe.

c. F

d. T

e. F—This is not a practical method.

Q.2.5 **Concave lenses:**

    a. Are represented by a negative sign
    b. Make objects look larger
    c. Are used to correct hypermetropia
    d. Are heavier than convex lenses
    e. Must always be made of plastic

Q.2.6 **Acquired hypermetropia is found in:**

    a. Aphakia
    b. Macular oedema
    c. Uncontrolled diabetes
    d. Retinitis pigmentosa
    e. Old age

The Watering Eye

Q.2.7 **Lacrimal obstruction:**

    a. Lacrimal obstruction usually occurs at the common canaliculus in children
    b. Entropion may be due to facial palsy
    c. Lacrimal obstruction in infants never resolves spontaneously
    d. Actinomycosis infection may cause lacrimal obstruction
    e. Buphthalmos is a cause of epiphora in infancy

Q.2.8 **In a child with a watery eye from birth:**

    a. Congenital glaucoma should be excluded
    b. Probing of the tear passages should be performed at 3 months of age
    c. The condition will not resolve spontaneously
    d. Antibiotic drops should be used continuously
    e. The nasolacrimal duct may be occluded at its lower end

For answers see over

Answers

A.2.5
  a. T
  b. F
  c. F
  d. F
  e. F

A.2.6
  a. T
  b. T
  c. F
  d. F—Myopia is more common in retinitis pigmentosa than in the normal population.
  e. F

A.2.7
  a. F—Lacrimal obstruction in children is usually at the lower end of the nasolacrimal duct.
  b. F—Facial palsy causes ectropion.
  c. F—Many cases resolve spontaneously in the first nine months.
  d. T—The organism resides in and obstructs the canaliculi.
  e. T—Photophobia and epiphora are features of congenital glaucoma.

A.2.8
  a. T—Congenital glaucoma may be present from birth.
  b. F—Time should be given to allow spontaneous resolution.
  c. F—Congenital obstruction of the nasolacrimal duct resolves spontaneously in most cases.
  d. F—Antibiotics should be reserved for acute infections.
  e. T

Q.2.9   Eversion of the lacrimal punctum:

a. Causes a dry eye problem
b. Can be cured by retropunctal cautery
c. Can be treated in the outpatient department
d. Is often bilateral
e. Is associated with entropion

Q.2.10   The following are important causes of a watering eye:

a. Epiphora
b. Ingrowing eyelashes
c. Corneal foreign body
d. Sarcoidosis
e. Late stage trachoma

The Dry Eye

Q.2.11   Dry eye and the tear film:

a. Dry eye is detected by Sjögren's test
b. Dry eye is associated with sarcoidosis
c. The anterior layer of the tear film contains mucin
d. Meibomian gland hyposecretion causes filamentary keratoconjunctivitis
e. "Dry eye" is a cause of epiphora

Q.2.12   The dry eye syndrome:

a. Is more common in warm weather
b. Is characterised by keratoconjunctivitis sicca
c. Is usually due to excessive drainage of tears
d. Should always be treated with local steroids
e. Should raise the suspicion of systematic disease

For answers see over

Answers

A.2.9   a. F
       b. T
       c. T
       d. T
       e. F

A.2.10   a. F—This *means* a watering eye.
        b. T
        c. T
        d. F—This is an uncommon cause of dry eye.
        e. F—Trachoma in its late stages causes dry eye problems.

A.2.11   a. F—Schirmer's test is one of the tests for a dry eye.
        b. T—This is a cause of dry eye in younger patients.
        c. F—The tear film consists of an anterior lipid layer, a central aqueous layer and a posterior mucin layer.
        d. F—Filament formation is associated with deficiency of the aqueous layer.
        e. T—Overflow of tears may occur with abnormalities of the tear film when there is normal reflex tear secretion.

A.2.12   a. F
        b. T
        c. F
        d. F
        e. T—Especially rheumatoid arthritis and sarcoidosis.

Lid Deformities

Q.2.13 Common eyelid deformities:

   a. Surgical treatment of ectropion is unsatisfactory
   b. A Meibomian cyst is a type of stye
   c. Spastic entropion is more common in the elderly
   d. Ptosis is caused by VIIth cranial nerve palsy
   e. A coloboma of the lid is a congenital deformity

Q.2.14 Ptosis:

   a. A 2 mm ptosis may be present in a complete IIIrd cranial nerve palsy
   b. May be induced by a Meibomian cyst
   c. May be relieved by guanethidine drops
   d. May be a feature of myasthenia gravis
   e. May be corrected by a levator recession

Q.2.15 Epicanthus:

   a. Is seen normally in Mongolian races
   b. Is a cause of squint
   c. Usually requires surgical correction
   d. May be associated with ptosis
   e. Affects the lateral part of the eyelid

Q.2.16 Entropion:

   a. Is common in infancy
   b. Is due to herpes simplex infection
   c. Is a condition of the elderly
   d. Is cured by surgery
   e. Requires a general anaesthetic for correction

For answers see over

Answers

A.2.13 a. F
    b. F—A stye is an acute infection of the apocrine gland at the lash root.
    c. T—And should be corrected surgically to prevent corneal damage from the inturned lashes.
    d. F—The oculomotor nerve raises the upper lid. The facial nerve closes it.
    e. T—When applied to the eye a coloboma is any congenital fusion defect.

A.2.14 a. F—A total IIIrd cranial nerve palsy causes a complete ptosis.
    b. T—One of the many mechanical causes.
    c. F—Guanethidine eye drops may cause ptosis.
    d. T
    e. F—This would increase the degree of ptosis.

A.2.15 a. T
    b. F—It may give the false impression of squint.
    c. F—It usually resolves with growth of the face.
    d. T
    e. F—The term refers to a fold of skin across the inner canthus.

A.2.16 a. F—It is rare in infancy.
    b. F
    c. T
    d. T
    e. F

Q.2.17 Anatomy

a. The VIIth cranial nerve mediates elevation of the upper lid
b. The lacrimal canaliculi run horizontally from the puncta to the nasolacrimal duct
c. The lash roots lie anterior to the opening of the Meibomian glands
d. The Meibomian glands are embedded in cartilage
e. Ptosis is only slight in Horner's syndrome

Q.2.18 Eyelashes:

a. May grow irregularly following chronic lid infection
b. When ingrowing are usually removed by radiotherapy
c. Should be epilated in entropion
d. When ingrowing may be an indication for contact lens wear
e. Are normally found growing on the lacrimal caruncle

Q.2.19 Some conjunctival causes of red eye:

a. Subconjunctival haemorrhage is often indicative of a blood dyscrasia
b. Lacrimal obstruction is a cause of unilateral conjunctivitis
c. Adenoviral keratoconjunctivitis may cause visual impairment for many months
d. A conjunctival culture for bacteria is useful in chronic conjunctivitis
e. Vernal keratoconjunctivitis affects mainly the lower lids

Q.2.20 Blepharitis:

a. Is often due to a staphylococcal infection
b. Is more common in atopic subjects
c. Is associated with marginal corneal ulceration
d. Should be treated with long-term topical steroids
e. Is a common cause of red eye

For answers see over

Answers

A.2.17 a. F—It supplies orbicularis oculi.
          b. F—They have an initial short vertical course from the puncta then run horizontally and join to form the common canaliculus.
          c. T—But may rarely be congenital.
          d. F—They are embedded in the fibrous tarsal plate.
          e. T

A.2.18 a. T—Trichiasis may be used by longstanding blepharitis.
          b. F—Epilation by forceps, electrolysis or by cryotherapy are accepted methods.
          c. F—The entropion itself should be treated.
          d. T
          e. T

A.2.19 a. F—Subconjunctival haemorrhage is rarely due to this cause.
          b. T
          c. T—Subepithelial corneal infiltrates may persist for months.
          d. F—It is of little value in most cases.
          e. F—Vernal keratoconjunctivitis or spring catarrh is characterised by giant papillae under the upper lid.

A.2.20 a. T—Particularly in chronic blepharitis.
          b. T
          c. T
          d. F—These may be used in the short term but the dangers of long-term steroid therapy to the skin and eye preclude its continuous use.
          e. T

Lid Tumours

Q.2.21 **Some types of eyelid tumour:**
  a. Malignant melanoma is the commonest malignant tumour of the eyelid
  b. Xanthelasma begins to appear at the outer canthus
  c. Papillomata do not occur on the lid margin
  d. Capillary haemangioma is associated with glaucoma
  e. Molluscum contagiosum may cause conjunctivitis

Q.2.22 **More lid tumours and their management:**
  a. Lipoma is the commonest tumour of the eyelids
  b. Keratoacanthoma resembles a squamous carcinoma
  c. Meibomian cysts resolve spontaneously in 6–9 months
  d. All lumps in the eyelids should be biopsied
  e. Radiotherapy should be avoided for tumours on the eyelids

Conjunctiva and Cornea

Q.2.23 **Conjunctival red eye:**
  a. Subconjunctival haemorrhage is usually symptomless
  b. Pink eye is normally caused by Corynebacteria
  c. Chlamydial conjunctivitis does not respond to antibiotics
  d. Spring catarrh is associated with preauricular lymph-adenopathy
  e. Sensitivity to cleaning solutions may cause a red eye in contact-lens wearers

Q.2.24 **Pingueculum:**
  a. Is a premalignant condition of the conjunctiva
  b. Occurs in up to 25% of the normal population
  c. Requires surgical removal in the majority of cases
  d. Is a degenerative condition of the conjunctiva
  e. Can cause a disturbance in the tear film, leading to dry spots

For answers see over

Answers

A.2.21 a. F—Basal cell carcinoma is the commonest malignant tumour of the eyelids.
  b. F—These aggregations of lipid-swollen cells first appear at the inner canthus.
  c. F—Papillomata in this position often requires excision for cosmetic reasons.
  d. T—This is particularly so if the haemangioma is on the upper lid and the glaucoma may occur at any age.
  e. T—Should be considered particularly with uniocular conjunctivitis.

A.2.22 a. F—
  b. T—But it is benign and may resolve spontaneously.
  c. T—But incision and currettage can give prompt relief.
  d. T—In theory. In practice, obvious Meibomian cysts are not routinely biopsied.
  e. F—Adequate screening of the globe and lacrimal canaliculi is needed.

A.2.23 a. T—May be noticed after the patient has looked in a mirror.
  b. F—Acute purulent conjunctivitis is usually caused by the pneumococcus.
  c. F—Tetracycline is the treatment of choice.
  d. F—Preauricular lymphadenopathy is not a feature of allergic types of conjunctivitis.
  e. T—Preservatives in these solutions are usually the culprits.

A.2.24 a. F—It is an elastotic degeneration of the conjunctiva.
  b. T
  c. F—It is usually asymptomatic.
  d. T—See above.
  e. T—Symptoms of dry eye may develop in certain cases.

Q.2.25 Conjunctival pathology:

a. Pingueculum is best treated by radiotherapy
b. Conjunctival oedema is a feature of thyrotoxicosis
c. Tears are a good culture medium for bacteria
d. Conjunctival follicles specifically indicate viral conjunctivitis
e. Pterygia are more common in Australia than England

Q.2.26 Corneal inflammation and dystrophy:

a. Corneal pain is best treated by local anaesthetic drops
b. Marginal ulcers of the cornea are rare
c. Band degeneration is characterised by calcification in the posterior stroma of the cornea
d. Placido's disc is used in the diagnosis of keratoconus
e. Hard contact lenses are used in keratoconus

Q.2.27 Viral disease of the cornea and exposure keratitis:

a. Herpes simplex causes scarring of the cornea
b. Herpes simplex does not cause corneal anaesthesia
c. Dendritic ulcers should be treated with local steroids
d. Most cases of Bell's palsy require tarsorrhaphy
e. Post-herpetic neuralgia follows herpes zoster infection.

Q.2.28 Recurrent corneal abrasion:

a. Often occurs months after the original injury
b. Causes pain in the early morning on waking
c. Is due to infection
d. Responds to treatment with cocaine drops
e. Is usually evident to naked-eye examination

For answers see over

Answers

A.2.25 a. F—This mild degenerative condition of the paralimbal conjunctiva is common and usually symptomless, and thus may not require treatment.
b. T—Chemosis is another term for conjunctival oedema.
c. F—Tears contain antibacterial agents such as immunoglobulins and lysozyme.
d. F—A conjunctival follicle is a small germinal centre and is therefore a non-specific sign.
e. T—This condition is more common in hot, dry climates.

A.2.26 a. F—Under no circumstances should prolonged local anaesthetic drops be prescribed for any eye condition.
b. F—These are commonly found in staphyloccal blepharitis and are probably caused by a hypersensitivity to the exotoxin.
c. F—It is the anterior stromal layers that are affected in band degeneration.
d. T—This allows easy detection of the conical shape of the cornea in keratoconus.
e. T—These in effect provide a uniform refracting surface and may improve vision dramatically.

A.2.27 a. T—If the stroma is involved in the inflammatory process.
b. F.
c. F—The use of steroids on dendritic ulcers may have disasterous results.
d. F—Tarsorrhaphy is only usually required if the cornea is considered at risk of exposure.
e. T

A.2.28 a. T
b. T
c. F—It is due to instability of the epithelium.
d. F—These drops should be avoided.
e. F—The lesion has often healed by the time the patient sees the doctor and diagnosis depends on careful slit-lamp microscopy.

Q.2.29 Bacterial and viral infection of the cornea:

  a. Pain is a feature of late-stage herpes simplex keratitis
  b. Dendritic ulceration of the cornea is due to *Staphylococcus*
  c. Herpes simplex keratitis begins in the corneal epithelium and spreads to the stroma
  d. Corneal grafting should be avoided in herpes simplex infections of the cornea
  e. Marginal ulceration of the cornea is due to *Staphylococcus*

Q.2.30 The following are typical symptoms of allergic conjunctivitis:

  a. A mucopurulent discharge
  b. Markedly reduced vision
  c. Itching
  d. Watering
  e. Photophobia

Q.2.31 The following are causes of corneal oedema:

  a. Rubeotic glaucoma
  b. Herpes simplex keratitis
  c. Chalazia
  d. Fuch's endothelial dystrophy
  e. Intraocular implants

Q.2.32 In herpes zoster ophthalmicus:

  a. The condition is caused by an RNA virus
  b. Headache often precedes the rash
  c. The cornea can be rendered anaesthetic
  d. Glaucoma should be excluded
  e. An underlying malignancy is common

For answers see over

Answers

A.2.29
a. F—It is a feature of early infection but at a later stage the cornea becomes anaesthetic.
b. F—It is due to the herpes simplex virus.
c. T
d. F—Corneal grafting is occasionally indicated.
e. T—These common peripheral corneal infiltrates seen in elderly patients usually respond well to antibiotic drops.

A.2.30
a. F—This is found in infective conjunctivitis, particularly bacterial.
b. F
c. T—And is usually the cardinal symptom.
d. T
e. F—This will only occur in severe cases when the cornea is also involved.

A.2.31
a. T—Any cause of prolonged, severely raised intraocular pressure will cause corneal oedema.
b. T—As it is an inflammatory keratitis.
c. F
d. T—In this condition it is due to a progressive loss of the endothelial cells so necessary for the maintenance of corneal clarity.
e. T—Either by intermittent corneal touch or chronic inflammation reducing the endothelial cell count or, occasionally, glaucoma.

A.2.32
a. F—It is a double-stranded DNA virus.
b. T—The diagnosis is often not considered because of this in the early stages.
c. T—This may cause serious problems later.
d. T—An anterior uveitis or trabeculitis may cause acute or chronic raised pressure in these cases.
e. F—There is no evidence for this.

Q.2.33 Corneal oedema:

    a. Is a sign of thyrotoxicosis
    b. Causes the symptom of haloes round lights
    c. Is a specific sign of narrow angle glaucoma
    d. Is characterised by pain in the eye
    e. Is associated with damage to the corneal endothelium

Q.2.34 Corneal anaesthesia:

    a. May be due to damage to the maxillary division of the Vth cranial nerve
    b. Occurs after cataract surgery
    c. Is an early sign of acoustic neuroma
    d. Is a contraindication to ptosis surgery
    e. Is common after herpes zoster infection of the eye

Q.2.35 The following are causes of chronic vascular congestion of the conjunctiva:

    a. Long-term use of adrenaline drops
    b. Polycythaemia vera
    c. Excessive physical exertion
    d. Hypertension
    e. Acne rosacea

Q.2.36 Episcleritis:

    a. Is a common cause of red eye in the elderly
    b. Is a self-limiting condition of young adults
    c. Is associated with excess conjunctival discharge
    d. Responds to local antibiotics
    e. Means inflammation of the sclera

For answers see over

Answers

A.2.33 a. F—But conjunctival oedema is seen in thyrotoxicosis.
b. T
c. F—It is seen in a number of other eye conditions.
d. F—But longstanding corneal oedema may cause pain due to rupture of bullae.
e. T—The corneal endothelium is thought to maintain the normal cornea in a state of relative dehydration.

A.2.34 a. F—It is due to damage to the ophthalmic division of this nerve.
b. T—The corneal incision divides the nerves, producing a wedge of temporary anaesthesia.
c. T—Tumours of the cerebellopontine angle may cause early Vth cranial nerve damage.
d. T—Surgical elevation of the lid leads to exposure keratitis in these cases.
e. T

A.2.35 a. T
b. T
c. F
d. F
e. T

A.2.36 a. F—It is more common in young adults.
b. T
c. F—The conjunctiva itself is not involved and hence there is no discharge.
d. F
e. F—The episclera is the layer of connective tissue between the conjunctiva and the sclera.

Red Painless Eye

Q.2.37 **Pain like visual impairment is an important symptom which helps in the diagnosis of the red eye. It often indicates a more serious problem. Consider the following:**

  a. Chronic conjunctivitis is normally due to bacterial infection
  b. Episcleritis is a complication of acute conjunctivitis
  c. Acute conjunctivitis should always be treated with antibiotics
  d. Refractive error is associated with chronic conjunctivitis
  e. Non-accidental injury is a cause of subconjunctival haemorrhage

Red Painful Eye

Q.2.38 **Iritis and acute angle closure glaucoma:**

  a. Iritis presents with severe pain and a small pupil
  b. Iritis is not the same as acute anterior uveitis
  c. Acute angle closure glaucoma is more common in myopes
  d. Acute angle closure glaucoma is a major cause of blindless
  e. The pupil is usually mid-dilated in acute angle closure glaucoma

Q.2.39 **The following cause a red painful eye with visual impairment:**

  a. Migraine
  b. Choroiditis
  c. Acute iridocyclitis
  d. Herpes simplex keratitis
  e. Optic neuritis

For answers see over

Answers

A.2.37 a. F—Unless there is associated lacrimal obstruction.
b. F—Episcleritis is a localised inflammation on the episclera and is not usually associated with infection.
c. F—It may not be bacterial in origin.
d. T—Constant rubbing of the eyes to improve the vision is only one of the mechanisms by which refractive errors may cause chronic conjunctivitis.
e. T—Bilateral subconjunctival haemorrhages in a child should always suggest non-accidental injury.

A.2.38 a. T—Ciliary and iris spasm causes a small pupil and severe pain.
b. T—Strictly speaking "anterior uveitis" refers to inflammation of the iris and ciliary body, that is, "iridocyclitis".
c. F—Myopic patients have deep anterior chambers and therefore are not at risk of acute glaucoma.
d. F—Acute glaucoma is much less common than chronic simple glaucoma, which is a major cause of blindness in the Western world.
e. T—There will usually be corneal oedema and a non-reactive mid-dilated pupil rendering the condition relatively easy to diagnose.

A.2.39 a. F—But migraine may be associated with conjunctival congestion.
b. F—This is a cause of visual impairment in a white eye.
c. T
d. T
e. F—A cause of sudden unilateral visual loss in young adults. The eye remains white. An afferent pupil defect is the important sign.

Failing Vision in Normal-Looking Eye

Q.2.40 **Some causes of visual failure in an eye which looks normal externally:**

a. Amblyopia of disuse is not treatable over the age of 6 years
b. Sympathetic ophthalmia occurs in Horner's syndrome
c. Diabetic control bears no relation to the advance of retinopathy
d. Cataract surgery may be carried out effectively in patients over 100 years old
e. In sphenoid wing meningiomas, loss of vision is usually the first symptom

Q.2.41 **In retinitis pigmentosa:**

a. Central vision is affected early
b. Night blindness occurs before reading difficulties
c. Cataract extraction may improve visual function
d. The dominantly inherited form is the most severe
e. Myopia is common

Q.2.42 **The following cause visual impairment in a white eye:**

a. Anterior uveitis
b. Senile macular degeneration
c. Cavernous sinus thrombosis
d. Retinitis pigmentosa
e. Presbyopia

Q.2.43 **The following are treatable causes of failing vision:**

a. Acute dacryocystitis
b. Chronic simple glaucoma
c. Retinitis pigmentosa
d. Trachoma
e. Hypertensive retinopathy

For answers see over

Answers

A.2.40 a. F—The vision in an amblyopic eye may improve with treatment up to the age of 9 or 10 years.

b. F—Sympathetic ophthalmia should not be confused with Horner's syndrome, due to a loss of sympathetic innervation to the eye.

c. F—Recent studies have shown that good diabetic control in the early stages may delay the appearance and progress of diabetic retinopathy.

d. T—There is no upper age limit in cataract surgery.

e. T—Because of their slowly growing nature, optic nerve compression and resulting loss of vision is usually the first symptom of these tumours.

A.2.41 a. F—Peripheral visual fields are affected first.

b. T—Rod function is impaired before cone function.

c. T—Retinitis pigmentosa is associated with a posterior subcapsular cataract.

d. F—The autosomal recessive form, followed by the X-linked recessive.

e. T

A.2.42 a. F—This is the same as iridocyclitis.

b. T

c. F—This is associated with conjunctival congestion and proptosis.

d. T—The patient notices impaired night vision in the early stages.

e. T—A common cause of blurred reading vision in middle age.

A.2.43 a. F—Does not cause loss of vision.

b. T

c. F—There is no known effective treatment at present.

d. T—Responds to tetracycline.

e. T—Vision and retinopathy improve with treatment of blood pressure.

Q.2.44 The following are untreatable causes of failing vision:

   a. Senile macular degeneration
   b. Myopic degeneration
   c. Optic neuritis
   d. Retinoblastoma
   e. Vitreous haemorrhage

Headache

Q.2.45 Some types of headache:

   a. Migraine sufferers see recurrent flashes of light in their peripheral fields
   b. Anaemic patients tend not to suffer from headache
   c. The headache of raised intracranial pressure is worse in the evenings
   d. Migraine may be associated with ophthalmoplegia
   e. Pituitary apoplexy is a neurosurgical emergency

Q.2.46 Some causes of headache:

   a. Cluster headaches follow herpes zoster infection
   b. Uncorrected refractive error does not cause headache
   c. Temporal arteritis may need one or more artery biopsies for diagnosis
   d. Vertical muscle imbalance is not a treatable cause of headache
   e. Overcorrected myopia causes headache

Q.2.47 The following usually present with headache:

   a. Chronic simple glaucoma
   b. Migraine
   c. Malignant melanoma of the choroid
   d. Acute frontal sinusitis
   e. Ocular torticollis

For answers see over

Answers

A.2.44 a. T—But treatment can alter the rate of progress in some carefully selected cases.
   b. T
   c. T—But the condition tends to recover spontaneously over 2 or 3 months.
   d. F—Retinoblastoma can be treated by radiotherapy and chemotherapy in some instances.
   e. F—Usually clears spontaneously but may be removed by vitrectomy if persists more than 6 months.

A.2.45 a. F—The scintillating scotoma of migraine is usually paracentral.
   b. F—On the contrary, headache may have many origins in the anaemic patient.
   c. F—Raised intracranial pressure characteristically causes a headache present on waking which improves as the day goes on.
   d. T—The IIIrd cranial nerve is the commonest nerve affected, and this condition occurs particularly in children.
   e. T

A.2.46 a. F—No association has been found between cluster headaches and herpes zoster.
   b. F—A refractive error should be ruled out in cases of persistent frontal headache or an aching sensation in the eyes.
   c. T—A positive biopsy is diagnostic but a negative biopsy does not exclude the condition.
   d. F—Treatment will consist of either prismatic spectacles or squint surgery.
   e. T—The constant accommodation required from spectacles that are too strong will cause headache in many patients.

A.2.47 a. F—Headache is not a feature of this type of glaucoma.
   b. T
   c. F
   d. T
   e. F—Refers to the head tilt seen in children with a vertical squint.

Q.2.48 **Headache and vomiting are features of:**

a. Raised intracranial pressure
b. Migraine
c. Acute narrow angle glaucoma
d. Acute iridocyclitis
e. Incomitant squint

Q.2.49 **The routine investigation of headache should include:**

a. Computer-aided tomography scan
b. Lumbar puncture
c. Measurement of erythrocyte sedimentation rate
d. Measurement of blood pressure
e. Hess chart

Q.2.50 **The following types of headache usually have a physical basis and a positive outcome to investigations:**

a. Tenderness of the scalp when brushing the hair
b. Pain like a red hot needle through the skull
c. Bursting sensation worse on bending
d. Pain radiating from the back of the head with neck movement
e. Frontal headache after a day's work

Contact Lenses

Q.2.51 **The following may result from contact lens wear:**

a. Conical cornea
b. Follicular conjunctivitis
c. Corneal vascularisation
d. Angular conjunctivitis
e. Subconjunctival haemorrhages

For answers see over

Answers

A.2.48 a. T—Together with papilloedema.
          b. T—Vomiting may follow the headache.
          c. T—Has been mistaken for an acute abdomen.
          d. F
          e. F—Unless associated with raised intracranial pressure.

A.2.49 a. F—This investigation should be reserved for cases where an intracranial space-taking lesion is suspected.
          b. F—Reserved for cases with a suspected neurological cause.
          c. T—Especially to exclude temporal arteritis in the elderly.
          d. T
          e. F—But may be indicated if an ocular muscle imbalance is suspected as the cause.

A.2.50 a. T—In the elderly patient with temporal arteritis.
          b. F—This type of pain often has no detectable cause.
          c. T—The headache of raised intracranial pressure may be described like this.
          d. T—This type of headache is associated with cervical spondylosis.
          e. F—A common type of headache where a physical cause may not be found.

A.2.51 a. F—This is an inherited corneal dystrophy but it should be mentioned that some authorities have claimed that contact lenses may be a cause.
          b. T—May be a persistent problem in contact-lens wearers.
          c. T—Seen sometimes in long-term wearers.
          d. F
          e. F—A common condition which is not a particular feature of contact-lens wear.

Q.2.52   Some indications and contraindications:

   a. Contact lenses retard the progress of myopia
   b. Contact lenses are most useful when refractive error is large
   c. The commonest complication of wearing contact lenses is anterior uveitis
   d. Contact lenses are useful in presbyopia
   e. Hard contact lenses are more effective than soft contact lenses in correcting astigmatism

Q.2.53   Contact lenses should be avoided in:

   a. Patients with hay fever
   b. Patients who require regular eye drops
   c. Emmetropic patients
   d. Unilateral aphakia
   e. Elderly patients

For answers see over

Answers

A.2.52 a. F—There is no scientific evidence for this.
  b. T—High-powered spectacle lenses pose many problems for patients.
  c. F—A mild conjunctivitis is the commonest complication of contact-lens wear.
  d. F—Although bifocal contact lenses exist, most patients prefer spectacles.
  e. T—A soft contact lens will only reflect the underlying corneal curvature and therefore not correct degrees of astigmatism over 1 dioptre.

A.2.53 a. F—But hay fever may be a cause of intolerance.
  b. F—Except in the case of soft lenses.
  c. F—Emmetropia means no refractive error but contact lenses are also used for protective purposes.
  d. F—Unilateral aphakes can only use the eyes together if wearing a contact lens in the operated eye.
  e. T—Many elderly patients find it difficult to handle contact lenses. Long-term wear lenses may sometimes be indicated.

3 Problems of the Eye Surgeon

3. *Problems of the Eye Surgeon*

Cataract

Q.3.1 **Lens anatomy and ageing:**
  a. The epithelium of the lens covers the anterior surface only
  b. The lens capsule covers the anterior surface only
  c. There is a "pigs tail"-like remnant of the hyaloid artery on the anterior surface of the lens
  d. Presbyopia is due to a weakening of the ciliary muscle in middle age
  e. Posterior subcapsular cataract reduces visual acuity earlier than does anterior subcapsular cataract

Q.3.2 **The human lens:**
  a. Gradually shrinks with age
  b. Receives its blood supply from the ciliary body
  c. Is held taut by a series of radial fibres
  d. Shows an increase in anterior/posterior diameter during accommodation
  e. Is enclosed by a single-layered epithelium

Q.3.3 **Lens anatomy and development:**
  a. The lens has no capsule
  b. Each lens fibre is a prismatic six-sided band
  c. Epithelial cells at the lens equator multiply to form lens fibres
  d. The lens is derived from mesodermal cells
  e. The lens has the same refractive index as the vitreous

Q.3.4 **Aetiology of cataract:**
  a. Cataract is due to failure to wear dark glasses
  b. Trauma is unlikely to cause cataract unless the eye is perforated
  c. Retinitis pigmentosa is associated with cataract
  d. Diabetic cataract begins in the anterior part of the lens
  e. Diabetic patients are more prone to senile cataract formation at an early age

For answers see over

Answers

A.3.1 a. T
  b. F—The lens capsule, of course, encompasses the whole lens.
  c. F—This is the Mittendorf's dot on the posterior surface of the lens.
  d. F—Presbyopia is due to decreasing elasticity of the lens.
  e. T—Opacities have more effect on vision if they are near an optical point known as the nodal point. This is positioned in the posterior part of the lens.

A.3.2 a. F—It grows slowly throughout life.
  b. F—It is avascular.
  c. T—It is held taut by the zonule.
  d. T
  e. F—There is an anterior epithelial layer only.

A.3.3. a. F
  b. T
  c. T
  d. F—Derived from ectoderm.
  e. F—The diminishing range of accommodation with age is probably due to lens sclerosis.

A.3.4 a. F—There is no clear evidence that increased exposure to sunlight hastens cataract formation.
  b. F—Blunt trauma can cause cataracts.
  c. T—Usually of the posterior subcapsular type.
  d. F—Acute diabetic cataract may begin in the anterior or posterior cortex of the lens
  e. T—This has been shown to be true statistically.

Q.3.5   Symptoms and signs of cataract:

a. Apparent kinking of straight lines is a symptom of cataract
b. Cataract patients often experience monocular diplopia
c. Cataracts are often painful
d. Reading vision is lost early in the progress of cataract formation
e. Cataract is a cause of an afferent pupil defect

Q.3.6   Management of cataract:

a. The early stages of cataract are not usually visible ophthalmoscopically
b. Aphakic patients are unable to wear contact lenses
c. Cataract surgery is reserved for those in whom medical treatment has failed
d. The pupil reaction is a useful index of retinal function in dense cataracts
e. Congenital cataract may show an autosomal dominant inheritance pattern

Q.3.7   Surgery of cataract:

a. An extracapsular cataract extraction involves leaving most of the lens capsule in situ
b. Cataract surgery has been performed for more than 300 years
c. Most cataracts in the UK are removed as a day case
d. Patients should remain off work for 3 months after cataract surgery
e. Glaucoma surgery may induce cataract formation

Q.3.8   In an intracapsular cataract extraction:

a. The posterior capsule is left behind
b. An iridectomy is always performed
c. Vitreous loss may occur
d. A posterior chamber implant can be inserted
e. The wound is usually placed laterally

For answers see over

Answers

A.3.5   a. F—This is usually a symptom of macula disease.
            b. T—Due to irregular defraction of light.
            c. F—They usually cause painless loss of vision.
            d. F—Early cataracts cause changes in distance acuity rather than reading acuity.
            e. F—This would indicate retinal or optic nerve damage.

A.3.6   a. T—But they may be seen with a slit lamp.
            b. F—Contact lenses may be used in aphakia.
            c. F—Medical treatment for cataracts is still at the experimental stage.
            d. T—Although it may still be normal in isolated macula disease.
            e. T

A.3.7   a. T—Only a portion of the anterior capsule is removed.
            b. T—It has been performed for more than 2000 years.
            c. F—Although this is now the case in the United States.
            d. F—This will depend on the individual patient.
            e. T

A.3.8   a. F—The lens is removed in toto.
            b. T—This is to prevent pupil block glaucoma.
            c. T—Surgical techniques are designed to prevent this occurring.
            d. F—There could be no support for such an implant.
            e. F—The superior limbus is used in most cases.

Q.3.9   Further surgical considerations:
  a. Intraocular implants are only used in long-sighted patients
  b. Cataract surgery is more successful if performed at an early stage
  c. Systemic steroids are used routinely during cataract surgery
  d. There is an increased risk of retinal detachment after cataract surgery
  e. Cataract surgery will only correct vision to 6/12

Q.3.10   A mature white cataract:
  a. Can develop rapidly overnight
  b. Will cause no perception of light
  c. Can be associated with retinoblastoma
  d. May lead to glaucoma
  e. Always requires removal

Q.3.11   In the management of cataract surgery:
  a. It is usual to operate on the better seeing eye first
  b. An inpatient stay of 10 days must be anticipated
  c. The patient is offered the choice of laser treatment
  d. The patient is expected to be out of bed on the first postoperative day
  e. It may be necessary to instill drops for several weeks postoperatively

Q.3.12   Intraocular implants:
  a. Usually have an optical strength of 19–21 dioptres
  b. Are more often positioned behind the iris
  c. Are sewn into the ciliary body
  d. Cause a severe rejection reaction unless suitable precautions are taken
  e. Prolong the period of inpatient stay

For answers see over

Answers

A.3.9 a. F—They may be used in emmetropic, myopic or hypermetropic patients.
        b. F—The density of the opacity has no bearing on the surgical results.
        c. F—Local steroids are usually postoperatively.
        d. T—Although this is less common with extracapsular extraction.
        e. F—A best corrected vision of 6/6 or better is not unusual, providing no other disease process is present.

A.3.10 a. T—In occasional circumstances.
        b. F—One can perceive light through closed lids if retina and optic nerve are functional.
        c. T
        d. T—By inflammatory or physical mechanisms.
        e. F—The decision will depend on the individual case.

A.3.11 a. F—The reverse is true.
        b. F—The hospitalisation will depend on the surgeon and the individual patient.
        c. F—At the present time laser treatment alone cannot treat cataracts.
        d. T—Modern surgical techniques have allowed this to be possible.
        e. T

A.3.12 a. T
        b. T
        c. F
        d. F—Polymethylmethacrylate, the material used, is biologically inert.
        e. F—The period of inpatient stay has been steadily diminishing in spite of the popularity of implants.

Q.3.13 The important complications after implant surgery are as follows:

a. Secondary glaucoma
b. Hyphaema
c. Opacification of the posterior lens capsule
d. Abnormally low intraocular pressure
e. Loss of binocular vision

Q.3.14 Cataracts are known to be associated with:

a. Galactosaemia
b. Longstanding facial palsy
c. Infrared radiation
d. Microwave ovens
e. Prolonged use of aspirin

Q.3.15 Opacities in the lens may take the form of:

a. Concentric rings
b. Cartwheel-like spokes in the cortex
c. Brown colouration of the nucleus
d. Opacification of the capsule only
e. Opacification of the lens sutures

Q.3.16 The following drugs are known to cause cataracts:

a. Sodium salicylate
b. Chlorpromazine
c. Epanutin
d. Systemically administered steroids
e. Quinine

For answers see over

Answers

A.3.13 a. T—But more often a transient problem in the immediate postoperative period.

         b. T—But bleeding into the anterior chamber is now rare except in diabetics.

         c. T—May occur in 25% of cases. Treatment entails opening the capsule with the Nd: YAG laser.

         d. F

         e. F

A.3.14 a. T

         b. F

         c. T

         d. F

         e. F

A.3.15 a. F

         b. T

         c. T

         d. F

         e. T

A.3.16 a. F

         b. T

         c. F

         d. T

         e. F

Glaucoma

Q.3.17 Aqueous formation:

  a. The normal intraocular pressure should be below 15 mmHg (2000 Pa)
  b. Aqueous veins carry blood to the vortex veins
  c. Aqueous is produced by passive diffusion from the ciliary body
  d. The intraocular pressure shows a diurnal variation
  e. Beta blocking agents delivered topically to the eye reduce aqueous formation

Q.3.18 Open angle glaucoma:

  a. Chronic open angle glaucoma is usually due to impaired drainage of aqueous
  b. Headache is a common symptom of open angle glaucoma
  c. The cardinal signs of chronic open angle glaucoma are field loss, impaired visual acuity and cupping of the disc
  d. Chronic glaucoma causes constriction of the pupil
  e. Chronic glaucoma is a cause of an afferent pupil defect

Q.3.19 Treatment:

  a. Oral beta blockers are the mainstay of glaucoma treatment
  b. Glaucoma in infants is a surgical problem
  c. Visual loss from glaucoma is irrecoverable
  d. Adrenalin should never be prescribed for chronic open angle glaucoma
  e. Acetazolamide (Diamox) increases aqueous outflow

Q.3.20 A trabeculectomy:

  a. Is a form of cataract operation
  b. May be indicated in angle closure glaucoma
  c. May be indicated in chronic simple glaucoma
  d. Involves cryotherapy to the ciliary body
  e. Involves excision of a section of choroid

For answers see over

A.3.17 a. F—A pressure below or equal to 21 mmHg is considered to be normal.

b. F—These carry blood to the episcleral veins.

c. F—There is an active component to aqueous production.

d. T—And this may explain a normal pressure reading in a glaucomatous eye.

e. T—There are now many examples on the market.

A.3.18 a. T—The site of dysfunction is thought to be the trabecular meshwork in most cases.

b. F—Only occasionally is this true.

c. F—Impaired visual acuity should be replaced by raised intraocular pressure and open angles on gonioscopy.

d. F

e. T—Especially in the later stages.

A.3.19 a. F—Beta blockers are delivered topically.

b. T—A high percentage of cases of congenital glaucoma are cured by goniotomy.

c. T—But some recovery is occasionally seen when a high intraocular pressure is made normal.

d. F—It is one of the treatment options.

e. F—This carbonic anhydrase inhibitor decreases aqueous production.

A.3.20 a. F

b. T—If the angle is sufficiently compromised by the attack.

c. T—This is the commonest surgical procedure performed for chronic simple glaucoma.

d. F—This would be cyclocryotherapy: a different procedure, sometimes used to reduce intraocular pressure.

e. F—It involves excision of a section of trabecular meshwork.

Q.3.21   Narrow angle glaucoma:

a. Acute angle closure glaucoma can lead to total blindness if untreated
b. Surgery in acute glaucoma is reserved for those cases not responding to medical treatment
c. Phenothiazines should be avoided in patients being treated for glaucoma
d. Narrow angle glaucoma is more common in the summer
e. Rubeotic glaucoma can occur following central retinal vein occlusion

Q.3.22   Secondary and congenital glaucoma:

a. Atropine should be avoided in the treatment of secondary glaucoma
b. Congenital glaucoma may be confused with lacrimal obstruction
c. Steroids cause a reduction in intraocular pressure in steroid responders
d. Herpes zoster of the eye usually causes painful secondary glaucoma
e. Glaucoma is a cause of amaurosis fugax

Q.3.23   The following may be found in glaucomatous discs:

a. A cup/disc ratio of less than 0.4
b. Pallor of the neural rim
c. Loss of disc capillaries
d. Disc haemorrhages
e. Nasal displacement of retinal vessels

Q.3.24   In cases of open angle glaucoma:

a. Diagnosis depends on the presence of cupping of the optic disc
b. The visual acuity must be carefully monitored
c. Haemorrhages by the optic disc may help in diagnosis
d. The upper half of the visual field tends to be affected first
e. Mydriatics should be avoided

For answers see over

Answers

A.3.21   a. T—Prompt referral and treatment are essential.
         b. F—Surgery is necessary in the vast majority of cases of acute narrow angle glaucoma.
         c. F—If the patient has had surgical treatment the slight mydriasis produced by phenothiazines is not a hazard.
         d. F—It is commoner during autumn and winter.
         e. T—Although it may be prevented by prophylactic photo-coagulation in susceptible cases.

A.3.22   a. F—This will depend on the aetiology of the secondary glaucoma.
         b. T—Both may cause a watering eye in infancy.
         c. F—An elevation.
         d. F—The secondary glaucoma tends to be painless.
         e. T—These attacks of transient loss of vision may occur when the pressure is fluctuating markedly.

A.3.23   a. F—The cup/disc ratio is usually greater than 0.6.
         b. T—Due to atrophy of the nerve fibres.
         c. T
         d. T—Occasional small haemorrhages are seen.
         e. T—As the cup enlarges.

A.3.24   a. F—But this is an important sign.
         b. F—The visual acuity may not be affected until an advanced stage of the disease.
         c. T
         d. T
         e. F—They may be used to inspect the fundus if the angle is open.

Q.3.25 Glaucomatous defects in the visual field:

a. May progress to blindness in a few months if left untreated
b. Follow the pattern of the retinal nerve fibres
c. May improve after drainage surgery
d. Cause symptoms at an early stage in the disease
e. Do not occur in the absence of raised intraocular pressure

Q.3.26 Narrow angle glaucoma:

a. Tends to have a seasonal incidence
b. Is best treated conservatively
c. Is usually cured by surgery
d. Causes a characteristic type of iris atrophy
e. Is due to an abnormality of the trabecular meshwork

Q.3.27 Intraocular pressure:

a. Is normally below 21 mm H_2O
b. Is often raised in patients with systemic hypertension
c. Is raised when the pupils are dilated in normal subjects
d. Becomes low when the retina is detached
e. Is raised by increasing venous pressure

Q.3.28 Secondary glaucoma:

a. May be associated with central retinal vein thrombosis
b. May be caused by malignant melanoma of the choroid
c. May complicate optic neuritis
d. Is treated in the same way as open angle glaucoma
e. May follow contusion injury of the eye

For answers see over

Answers

A.3.25 a. T
     b. T—This accounts for the characteristic arcuate scotoma.
     c. T—But this is not a common occurrence.
     d. F
     e. F—Seen in "low tension glaucoma".

A.3.26 a. T—It is more common in the autumn months.
     b. F—Requires surgery without delay.
     c. T
     d. T—Causes "whorl atrophy".
     e. F

A.3.27 a. F—Should be mmHg not H_2O.
     b. F—Only coincidentally.
     c. F
     d. T
     e. T

A.3.28 a. T
     b. T
     c. F
     d. F—The cause of glaucoma must be treated.
     e. T—Especially when there is recession of the angle of the anterior chamber.

Retinal Detachment

Q.3.29   Causes and incidence:

a. Retinal detachment is more common in elderly debilitated patients
b. Retinal detachment becomes bilateral in 1% of cases
c. The detached retina is separated from the choroid by fluid
d. After surgery for retinal detachment the visual field is usually largely restored in 2–3 days
e. Renal failure can cause retinal detachment

Q.3.30   Preoperative assessment:

a. Retinal detachment usually occurs without warning symptoms
b. Malignant melanoma of the choroid may present as a detached retina
c. The retina is best repositioned by laser treatment
d. Retinal detachment is more common in hypermetropic patients
e. Inferior nasal retinal detachment causes superotemporal field loss

Q.3.31   Management:

a. Retinal detachment can be prevented by prophylactic treatment
b. Zigzagging flashes across the central field is a common symptom of retinal detachment
c. Detached retina can be replaced by a retinal transplant
d. Retina surgery is ineffective if the retina has been detached for more than 2 months
e. Visual acuity return following retinal detachment may improve up to 18 months following surgery

For answers see over

Answers

A.3.29 a. F—They are most common in late middle age.
  b. F—It is bilateral in 10% of cases.
  c. F—The fluid is between sensory retina and pigment epithelium.
  d. T
  e. T—This is one of the causes of serous detachment.

A.3.30 a. F—"Flashes and floaters" are common warning symptoms.
  b. T
  c. F—The laser may be used for sealing flat retinal breaks but is of little use once the retina has detached.
  d. F—It is more common in myopes.
  e. T

A.3.31 a. T
  b. F—They are usually in the peripheral field.
  c. F—One cannot transplant central nervous tissue in humans at present.
  d. F—Peripheral retina may regain its function after surgery if it has been detached for many months.
  e. T

Questions

Q.3.32 Traumatic retinal detachment:

a. Is a recognised boxing injury
b. May be delayed for some months following injury
c. Only occurs in susceptible individuals
d. Is a surgical emergency
e. Is always due to holes in the retina

Q.3.33 The following symptoms are typical of retinal detachment:

a. A dark shadow across the field of vision
b. Seeing flashing lights on bending the neck
c. Monocular diplopiae
d. Rapid deterioration of reading vision when aged 45 years
e. Black spots in front of the eyes

Q.3.34 Vitreous detachment:

a. Is a common change in middle age
b. Is usually of no pathological significance
c. May initiate a retinal detachment
d. Requires surgical replacement
e. May cause the symptom "flashes and floaters"

Q.3.35 Choroidal detachment

a. Is the same as retinal detachment
b. Is common in the immediate postoperative period after cataract surgery
c. Means separation of the choroid from the sclera
d. Often resolves spontaneously
e. Is associated with raised intraocular pressure

Q.3.36 Retinal detachment may be caused by:

a. Rapid eye movements
b. Peripheral retinal degeneration
c. Eclampsia
d. Diabetic retinopathy
e. Vitamin A deficiency

For answers see over

Answers

A.3.32 a. T
          b. T
          c. F
          d. T—But surgery may sometimes be delayed in longstanding cases.
          e. F—May be due to traction from fibrous bands in the vitreous.

A.3.33 a. T
          b. F—Flashes with neck movement are more often related to vertebrobasilar ischaemia.
          c. F
          d. F
          e. T—But these must be associated with flashes to be typical of premonitary symptoms.

A.3.34 a. T
          b. T
          c. T
          d. F
          e. T

A.3.35 a. F
          b. T
          c. T
          d. T
          e. F—Associated with ocular hypotonia.

A.3.36 a. F
          b. T
          c. T
          d. T
          e. F

Questions

Squint

Q.3.37 Some general considerations:

   a. Incomitant squint is more common in children
   b. Most squints recover by themselves
   c. Amblyopia of disuse is the commonest cause of unilateral impairment of vision in young adults
   d. Epicanthus is one of the musculofascial anomalies
   e. Birth trauma may cause a squint in the neonate

Q.3.38 The following are causes of squint in children:

   a. High myopia
   b. Epiphora
   c. Chronic uveitis
   d. Conjunctivitis
   e. Crouzon's anomaly

Q.3.39 The following are procedures which would correct a divergent squint:

   a. Medial rectus recession
   b. Lateral rectus recession
   c. Superior rectus resection
   d. Lateral rectus resection
   e. Inferior oblique recession

Q.3.40 In a recently acquired IVth nerve palsy:

   a. Diplopia is rare
   b. Diplopia may only be present when reading
   c. Closed head injury is a common cause
   d. Early surgery should be performed
   e. A head tilt is common

For answers see over

Answers

A.3.37 a. F—Concomitant squint is more common in children.
b. F—This is a common fallacy.
c. T
d. F—The folds of skin at the medial canthi give the misleading impression of a squint.
e. T

A.3.38 a. T—Particularly if unilateral.
b. F
c. T—Any media opacity may cause a squint.
d. F
e. T—This is one of the craniofacial anomalies.

A.3.39 a. F—This would make it worse.
b. T
c. F—This would induce a vertical squint.
d. F—This would make it worse.
e. F—The inferior oblique is primarily an elevator of the globe.

A.3.40 a. F
b. T
c. T—A bilateral IVth nerve palsy may follow severe head injury.
d. F—Surgery should be delayed until the condition is stable.
e. T—Chin down to the shoulder opposite the side of the lesion.

Q.3.41 Squints in childhood:

a. The parent may choose between surgery and the wearing of glasses for the management of their child's concomitant squint
b. Divergence excess squints in children are worse when viewing distant objects
c. Squints in children are not usually inherited
d. Double vision is a common presenting feature of childhood squint
e. IVth nerve palsy gives diplopia which is worse when reading

Q.3.42 The following are causes of vertical diplopia:

a. Dysthyroid eye disease
b. VIth nerve palsy
c. Blow-out fracture of the orbital floor
d. Cataract
e. Retinal detachment surgery

Q.3.43 Binocular vision and squint:

a. Fresnel prisms are used to treat adult squints
b. Latent squints are symptomless
c. The Maddox rod is used to measure the range of accommodation
d. Diplopia is rare in squint due to thyrotoxic eye disease
e. VIth nerve palsy is an important sign in raised intracranial pressure

Q.3.44 During a cover test on a right convergent squint in a child:

a. The right eye will converge when the left is covered
b. The left eye will diverge when the right is covered
c. The right eye will diverge when the left is covered
d. The left eye will converge when the right is covered
e. No movement of either eye will occur if eccentric fixation has developed

For answers see over

Answers

A.3.41 a. F
b. T—The child may need to be encouraged to look into the far distance to demonstrate this.
c. F—A dominant pattern of inheritance is often found.
d. F—Suppression of the squinting eye occurs leading to amblyopia.
e. T—The superior oblique muscle is the main depressor in adduction.

A.3.42 a. T—Associated with tethering of the inferior rectus muscle.
b. F—This causes horizontal diplopia.
c. T—Due to entrapment of inferior rectus or its check ligaments.
d. T—A cause of monocular diplopia.
e. T—Due to damage of elevators or depressors during the surgical procedure.

A.3.43 a. T—Particularly when a change in angle is expected or the patient is elderly and debilitated.
b. F—They often cause intermittent diplopia.
c. F—This device measures the angle of deviation of the eyes.
d. F—Diplopia is usually present in these cases.
e. T—This is thought to be due to pressure on the nerve as it crosses the tentorium.

A.3.44 a. F
b. F—The child is already fixing with the left eye.
c. T—To take up fixation.
d. F—See (b) above.
e. T—The right eye will use an extrafoveal point for fixation even when the left eye is covered.

Q.3.45 In an accommodative squint:

a. The eyes are usually myopic
b. The angle of squint is greater for near fixation when the patient is not wearing glasses
c. A full correction should be prescribed for the optical error
d. Bifocals may be used in children
e. The squint is usually divergent

Q.3.46 In an amblyopic eye:

a. Single letters are read better than lines of letters
b. The acuity will be improved by patching the fellow eye after the age of 8 years
c. Optic atrophy will develop in time
d. The pupil reactions will be normal
e. The peripheral visual fields will be constricted

Tumours of the Eye

Q.3.47 Malignant tumours of the globe:

a. Malignant melanoma of the choroid metastasises early
b. Retinoblastoma is usually recessively inherited
c. Most treated retinoblastoma patients survive into adult life
d. Melanoma of the iris is very malignant
e. Conjunctival melanoma is very malignant

Q.3.48 Dermoid cysts in the orbit:

a. Are most common in the inferior medial quadrant
b. Are highly malignant tumours
c. Are rarely fixed to bone
d. Usually present as solid craggy masses
e. Do not show on X-rays or computer-aided tomography scans

For answers see over

Answers

A.3.45 a. F—They are usually hypermetropic.
          b. T—As accommodation is linked to convergence.
          c. T—To allow full correction of the squint.
          d. T
          e. F—It is convergent.

A.3.46 a. T—The crowding phenomenon.
          b. F—Only in rare circumstances is this the case.
          c. F—An amblyopic eye is normal to ophthalmoscopic examination.
          d. T
          e. F—Thus an amblyopic eye may be very valuable to the patient even with low central acuity.

A.3.47 a. F—This usually occurs when the tumour has grown to a size greater than 10 mm in diameter.
          b. F—50% of retinoblastomata are dominantly inherited.
          c. T
          d. F—It carries an excellent prognosis if treated early.
          e. T—Early diagnosis and treatment is mandatory.

A.3.48 a. F—The upper outer quadrant.
          b. F—They are hamartomas.
          c. F—This should be determined prior to surgery.
          d. F—They are usually smooth fluctuant lesions.
          e. F—These may show posterior extension of the lesion and fixation to bone.

Q.3.49 Lid tumours:

a. Most strawberry naevi in infancy regress spontaneously
b. Basal cell carcinoma is rare on the eyelids
c. Keratoacanthoma is a rare malignant tumour of the eyelids
d. Squamous cell carcinomata of the eyelids rarely involve local lymph nodes
e. Basal cell carcinoma is a radiosensitive tumour

Q.3.50 A rhabdomyosarcoma:

a. Rarely causes proptosis
b. Is commonest in older adults
c. May be misdiagnosed as orbital cellulitis
d. Is a tumour of smooth muscle cells
e. Is a highly malignant tumour

Q.3.51 Proptosis and enophthalmos:

a. Proptosis is due to spasm of the eyelids
b. Proptosis is commonly caused by thyrotoxic eye disease
c. Lacrimal tumours do not usually present with proptosis
d. Orbital cellulitis is usually secondary to intraocular infection
e. Enophthalmos occurs with blow-out fractures of the orbit

Q.3.52 The following are causes of proptosis:

a. Caroticocavernous fistula
b. Frontal sinus mucocele
c. Cachexia
d. Optic nerve glioma
e. IIIrd nerve palsy

For answers see over

Answers

A.3.49 a. T—They only require treatment if their physical position induces a risk of amblyopia.
  b. F—The eyelid is a common site for these tumours.
  c. F—This is a benign lesion.
  d. F
  e. T

A.3.50 a. F—Proptosis is invariably present.
  b. F—It is a tumour found almost exclusively in children.
  c. T—Growth may be very rapid with lid and conjunctival oedema.
  d. F—The diagnosis is confirmed by finding striations in the tumour cells on microscopy.
  e. T

A.3.51 a. F
  b. T—This is the commonest cause of unilateral or bilateral proptosis.
  c. F—They usually displace the globe forwards downwards and medially.
  d. F
  e. T—This is associated with herniation of orbital tissue through the fractured orbital floor.

A.3.52 a. T—Increased orbital blood volume.
  b. T—The eye is displaced forwards and downwards.
  c. F—Enophthalmos is common as orbital fat atrophies.
  d. T—An axial proptosis occurs.
  e. T—A mild proptosis occurs due to lack of tone in the rectus muscles.

Ocular Trauma

Q.3.53   Contusion injuries:

   a. Iridodonesis is associated with traumatic dislocation of the lens

   b. Optic atrophy may be an immediate complication of ocular contusion

   c. Sympathetic ophthalmia is more common after contusion injuries

   d. Secondary intraocular bleeding is a complication of hyphaema

   e. Retinal detachment may occur following blunt or penetrating trauma

Q.3.54   A patient with a corneal foreign body:

   a. Should be admitted to hospital for treatment

   b. Should be given systemic antibiotics

   c. Should have the foreign body removed in theatre

   d. Should have local antibiotics after removal

   e. Requires a pad on the eye for 7 days following removal

Q.3.55   Penetrating injuries:

   a. The rarity of infection after perforating injuries of the eye is due to protection from the vitreous

   b. Penetrating injuries of the eye demand urgent surgical repair

   c. Acetazolamide should be avoided in cases of penetrating injury

   d. Once the globe has been perforated the sight of the eye is inevitably lost

   e. Siderosis occurs following a retained ferrous intraocular foreign body

For answers see over

Answers

A.3.53 a. T—It is due to rupture of the zonule.
   b. F—Optic atrophy usually takes a few weeks to develop.
   c. F—It is more common after penetrating injuries involving incarceration of uveal tissue or retina.
   d. T—This occurs in between 5% and 10% of cases in the UK.
   e. T—The result of retinal tears or dialyses.

A.3.54 a. F—This is the commonest ocular injury presenting to an eye casualty!
   b. F—Unless perforation is suspected.
   c. F—Most can be removed in the outpatient treatment room using a loupe or at the slit lamp.
   d. T
   e. F—Most are healed within 24–48 hours.

A.3.55 a. F—The use of antibiotics has changed the prognosis in these cases.
   b. T—Delay increases the risk of infection.
   c. F—There is no particular contraindication to its use in these cases.
   d. F—Excellent visual results are often achieved with modern surgical techniques.
   e. T—A missed intraocular foreign body is a common cause of medicolegal litigation.

Q.3.56 Following a chemical injury to the eye:

a. Copious irrigation of the eye with water should be advised as first aid
b. When transferred to hospital an alkali should be used if an acid caused the injury
c. Corneal stromal oedema is a bad prognostic sign
d. Colliquative necrosis occurs with alkaline burns
e. Symblepharon may occur

Q.3.57 Hyphaema:

a. Means pus in the anterior chamber
b. Is a sure indication of previous contusion injury
c. May be followed by more serious complications after 2 days
d. Is a potential surgical problem
e. Is best treated by drainage in the outpatient department

Q.3.58 Intraocular foreign bodies:

a. If metallic, can be removed with a magnet
b. If glass, may be left in situ
c. If plastic, may show as radiolucent or radiodense in computer-aided tomography scans
d. If organic, are usually infected
e. If small and metallic, are usually sterile

Q.3.59 Contusion of the globe:

a. Usually affects the upper part of the eye
b. Is a cause of a fixed dilated pupil
c. Produces radial tears in the iris sphincter
d. Is not associated with glaucoma
e. Can cause recession of the angle of the anterior chamber

Q.3.60 Eyelid injuries:

a. No graft is required if half of the upper eyelid is lost
b. No graft is required if 25% of the lower lid is lost
c. Epiphora is the rule if the upper cannaliculus is severed
d. Are best closed with full thickness sutures at the lid margin
e. Tissue is usually lost following road traffic accidents

For answers see over

Answers

A.3.56 a. T—Normal saline may be substituted when the patient is hospitalised.
b. F—This may cause more damage than the original injury.
c. T—As is the degree of limbal ischaemia.
d. T—The noxious material is thus able to penetrate further into the tissues.
e. T—Measures should be taken to prevent this.

A.3.57 a. F—This is a hypopion.
b. F—This may occur spontaneously.
c. T—The main complication being secondary haemorrhage.
d. T—If the hyphaema causes secondary glaucoma and medical measures fail to control the pressure then surgical removal may be needed.
e. F—Under no circumstances.

A.3.58 a. F—*Magnetic* foreign bodies may be removed with a magnet if it is thought prudent to do so.
b. T—Depending on their position and the nature of the injury.
c. T—Depending on the plastic.
d. T—These require urgent removal and high dose local and systemic antibiotics.
e. T—They are heat sterilised when formed.

A.3.59 a. F—The lower outer part of the eye is most vulnerable.
b. T—This would be traumatic mydriasis.
c. T—These may interfere with pupillary constriction.
d. F
e. T—This is one of the causes of glaucoma.

A.3.60 a. F—If over one third of the upper lid is lost a graft is inevitably required.
b. T—Direct closure is usually possible here.
c. F—The lower canaliculus carries the lion's share of the tears.
d. F—The lid margin should be sutured in at least two layers.
e. F—Tissue loss is rare in road traffic accidents although it may not appear so at first glance.

Q.3.61 Sympathetic ophthalmia:

a. Is a common sequel to perforating injuries
b. Leads to inflammation in the uninjured eye
c. Resists all medical treatment
d. Has a histological similarity to tuberculosis
e. Is due to excessive exposure to ultraviolet light

Q.3.62 Retinal burns:

a. May be caused by X-rays
b. Are associated with the drug LSD (lysergic acid diethylamide)
c. Can appear as macula holes after viewing eclipses
d. Are prevented by the use of overexposed film when sun gazing
e. Are found following snow blindness

Q.3.63 The following are signs of non-accidental injury in a child:

a. Retinal haemorrhage
b. Cataract
c. Subconjunctival haemorrhage
d. Retinoblastoma
e. Ocular albinism

Q.3.64 Radiation and chemical burns:

a. X-rays are focussed on to the retina by the optical media
b. Glassblower's cataract is due to exposure to ultraviolet light
c. Cataracts have been shown to be more common in patients who live close to nuclear power stations
d. Ultraviolet light causes punctate keratitis which usually resolves in 48 hours
e. Alkali burns tend to be associated with a poorer prognosis than acid burns

For answers see over

Answers

A.3.61 a. F—It is very rare.
b. T—Hence the name.
c. F—It usually responds to high-dose steroids.
d. T—The choroid is infiltrated with a granulomatous inflammatory response.
e. F

A.3.62 a. F—X-rays are not focussed by the eye but may cause retinal vascular damage in high doses.
b. T—Bilateral burns from sun gazing occurs.
c. T
d. F—This is not adequate protection.
e. F—This is ultraviolet damage which does not penetrate the cornea with sufficient energy to damage the retina.

A.3.63 a. T—These are rare in children unless caused by severe anaemia or trauma.
b. F—Blunt trauma.
c. T—Raised venous pressure from shaking, especially upside down.
d. F—There is no evidence for this.
e. F—This is inherited.

A.3.64 a. F—X-rays pass undeviated through the eye.
b. F—This is due to infra-red radiation.
c. F—High doses of microwaves can cause cataracts in experimental animals.
d. T—As seen in "welders arc" or snow blindness.
e. T—Alkalis cause necrosis beyond the region of infiltration by the toxic material.

4. *Problems of the Medical Ophthalmologist*

Q.4.1   A best corrected visual acuity of 6/24:

  a. Is compatible with reading newsprint
  b. May be improved by refraction
  c. Equates to reading the fourth line down on the Snellen chart
  d. Is compatible with a vitreous haemorrhage in the eye
  e. A normal eye can read the 6/24 line at 24 m from the chart

Q.4.2   The following charts measure visual acuity:

  a. The Landolt C
  b. The Illiterate E
  c. The Ishihara plates
  d. The Arden gratings
  e. The Amsler chart

Q.4.3   The optokinetic drum:

  a. Invokes optokinetic nystagmus and can be used to measure visual acuity
  b. Has horizontal stripes of black and white
  c. Is useful in the diagnosis of hysterical blindness and malingering
  d. Can be used in experimental animals
  e. Produces a loud sound as it rotates

Q.4.4.   The following are true in presbyopia:

  a. It occurs at a younger age in hot climates
  b. Loss of near acuity is more noticeable in low illumination
  c. A patient aged 50 years should require a 3 dioptre addition for reading
  d. A patient aged 80 years still has 8 dioptres of accommodation available
  e. It can be corrected with varifocal lenses

For answers see over

Answers

A.4.1   a. F
        b. F—Best corrected indicates optimal refraction.
        c. F—The third line.
        d. T—Depending on the density of the haemorrhage.
        e. T

A.4.2   a. T—The patient has to identify the position of the gap in the "C" which is almost a circle.
        b. T—The direction of the "E" is identified.
        c. F—These test colour vision.
        d. T—Although measuring contrast sensitivity these can measure acuity at high spatial frequencies.
        e. F—This identifies macula or paramacula abnormalities.

A.4.3   a. T—Using different sized stripes.
        b. F—They are vertically orientated.
        c. T—Although it can be overcome with effort.
        d. T—A useful research tool.
        e. F—!

A.4.4   a. T—Although the exact reason for this is obscure.
        b. T—If contrast is greater, acuity is improved.
        c. F—This does not encourage the patient to use the accommodation reserve.
        d. F—Only 1–2 dioptres remains at this age.
        e. T—These avoid some of the problems of bifocals but may create their own.

Q.4.5   A best corrected visual acuity of 6/12:

 a. Is normal in the elderly
 b. In an anatomically normal eye usually indicates amblyopia
 c. Would indicate that the eye cannot read newsprint
 d. Is better than a best corrected acuity of 6/9
 e. In a diabetic would indicate that fundoscopy is required

Q.4.6   Dark adaptometry:

 a. Is abnormal in vitamin C deficiency
 b. Is abnormal in vitamin A deficiency
 c. Is useful in the diagnosis of hysterical blindness
 d. Measures only rod recovery
 e. Is abnormal in retinitis pigmentosa

Q.4.7   Visual acuity:

 a. Is a measure of rod function in the eye
 b. Cannot be measured routinely in children under 6 years
 c. Provides a good assessment of navigational vision
 d. Must be measured with the patient wearing reading glasses
 e. Cannot be measured in dumb patients

Q.4.8   Refraction:

 a. Means bending of light rays when passing from one medium to another
 b. Refers to measuring a patient's optical correction
 c. Cannot be performed in infancy
 d. Is distressing for elderly patients
 e. Is not usually carried out in hospital

Q.4.9   Colour vision

 a. Is impaired in 8% of males
 b. Is a useful test of peripheral retinal function
 c. Must be normal in airline pilots
 d. Is affected early in diabetic retinopathy
 e. Can be tested with a Snellen chart

For answers see over

Answers

A.4.5 a. F—Loss of vision should never be simply attributed to old age.
      b. T
      c. F—One would need to test the near vision in order to ascertain the reading vision.
      d. F
      e. T—Diabetic maculopathy may be the cause of the acuity loss.

A.4.6 a. F
      b. T—This is common in developing countries in children on a poor diet.
      c. F—The success of the test relies on good patient co-operation.
      d. F—Cones recover in the first 5 min of the test.
      e. T—As would be expected in a rod/cone dystrophy.

A.4.7 a. F—Acuity is a measure of cone function.
      b. F—Many methods are available for the measurement of visual acuity in children.
      c. F—A patient with constricted visual fields could have good visual acuity and yet be unable to walk about without difficulty.
      d. F—Acuity is usually measured in the distance.
      e. F—Various matching tests can be used.

A.4.8 a. T
      b. T—The word is also used in this sense in ophthalmology.
      c. F
      d. F
      e. F—Refraction is an important part of the routine examination of an eye.

A.4.9 a. T—Most patients with colour vision defects show X-linked recessive inheritance.
      b. F—It tests central function.
      c. T
      d. T
      e. F

Q.4.10 The following instruments measure intraocular pressure:

a. The Schiotz tonometer
b. The Perkins tonometer
c. Placido's disc
d. The Hertel exophthalmometer
e. The Goldmann tonometer

Q.4.11 Testing vision: visual acuity, refractive error and muscle balance:

a. A pinhole will improve most reduced acuities secondary to optical error up to 6/9 or better
b. An aphakic eye with normal corrected acuity will be improved to 6/9 with a pinhole
c. A cylindrical lens corrects astigmatism
d. Keratoconus produces regular astigmatism
e. A Maddox Wing tests muscle balance at distance fixation

Q.4.12 The following conditions are more common in high myopia:

a. Chronic simple glaucoma
b. Acute angle closure glaucoma
c. Retinal detachments
d. Concomitant squint
e. Macular haemorrhage

Uveitis

Q.4.13 Terminology:

a. Iridocyclitis is synonymous with posterior uveitis
b. Iritis does not occur without choroiditis
c. Hypopion is a sign of anterior uveitis
d. The "ciliary flush" occurs following the use of steroids
e. Keratic precipitates are white cell accumulations on the corneal endothelium

For answers see over

Answers

A.4.10 a. T—This is less frequently used nowadays.

b. T—This is a useful accurate, hand-held instrument.

c. F—This is used to detect irregularity of the surface of the cornea.

d. F—This is used to detect and measure proptosis.

e. T—This is the most commonly used method for routine measurement of the intraocular pressure.

A.4.11 a. T—Hence its use.

b. F—Pinholes become less reliable in myopia or hypermetropia of more than 8 dioptres (or aphakia).

c. T—As it refracts light maximally in one meridian and not at all at 90° to this meridian.

d. F—It causes irregular astigmatism that cannot be fully corrected with spectacles.

e. F—It tests binocular muscle balance for near fixation.

A.4.12 a. T

b. F—Acute angle closure glaucoma is seen in hypermetropia and virtually never in myopia.

c. T

d. F—Concomitant squint is more common in hypermetropia.

e. T

A.4.13 a. F—Iridocyclitis is anterior uveitis.

b. F—Although choroiditis is usually accompanied by anterior uveitis.

c. T—A fluid level of white cells in the anterior chamber.

d. F—This is the limbal injection found in keratitis.

e. T—Usually abbreviated to KPs.

Q.4.14 Some facts about uveitis: true or false?

a. A chronic low grade uveitis occurs in Still's disease
b. Uveitis is more common in smokers
c. Iritis causes a constricted pupil
d. Posterior uveitis is often bilateral
e. Uveitis is more common following squint surgery

Q.4.15 Causes and effects of uveitis:

a. *Toxoplasmosis gondii* is carried by dogs
b. Toxoplasmic chorioretinitis is usually acquired in utero
c. Iris bombé causes angle closure in uveitis
d. Mutton fat keratic precipitates are common in the uveitis associated with HLA B27
e. Uveitis is associated with cataract

Q.4.16 The symptoms of acute anterior uveitis are:

a. Straight lines look bent
b. Pain in the eye
c. Impaired dark adaptation
d. Photophobia
e. Micropsia

Q.4.17 Hypopion may be seen in:

a. Endophthalmitis
b. Behçet's disease
c. Fungal corneal ulcer
d. Retinoblastoma
e. Horner's syndrome

Q.4.18 When managing a case of acute anterior uveitis:

a. Steroids should be avoided
b. Atropine is used to treat secondary glaucoma
c. Investigations for systemic disease are often negative
d. The patient should be admitted to hospital
e. Mydriasis is important

For answers see over

Answers

A.4.14 a. T
        b. F
        c. T—Treatment is aimed at dilating the pupil to prevent adhesions.
        d. T—But the condition may remain unilateral for many years.
        e. F

A.4.15 a. F—It is found in cats' faeces and conveyed by flies.
        b. T—Ocular involvement is extremely rare in acquired toxoplasmosis.
        c. T—This is an uncommon mechanism for secondary glaucoma.
        d. F—Mutton fat keratic precipitates are associated with granulomatous uveitis typically due to sarcoidosis and sympathetic ophthalmitis.
        e. T

A.4.16 a. F
        b. T
        c. F
        d. T
        e. F

A.4.17 a. T—When organisms may be found in the hypopion.
        b. T—A cause of sterile hypopion.
        c. T—This may be infective or reactive.
        d. T—Either tumour cells or reactive or both.
        e. F

A.4.18 a. F—Steroids are routinely used.
        b. T—And to relieve ciliary spasm.
        c. T—80% of cases may fail to have any associated systemic disease.
        d. F—Admission is usually only indicated if the disease is bilateral and the sight is threatened.
        e. T

Q.4.19 **The signs of acute anterior uveitis include:**

   a. Conjunctival follicles
   b. Corneal oedema
   c. A dilated pupil
   d. Posterior synecheae
   e. Iris bombé

Q.4.20 **Posterior uveitis:**

   a. Is known to be associated with toxoplasmosis
   b. Is an inflammation of the retina
   c. Is usually painless
   d. Is a feature of thyrotoxic eye disease
   e. Is usually due to staphylococcal infection

Q.4.21 **Anterior uveitis may cause the following:**

   a. Cataract
   b. Glaucoma
   c. Keratoconus
   d. Hypotony
   e. Choroidal melanoma

Q.4.22 **The symptoms of posterior ureitis that occur commonly are:**

   a. Blurred vision
   b. Floaters
   c. A red eye
   d. Diplopia
   e. Epiphora

For answers see over

A.4.19 a. F
          b. T—Due to endothelial dysfunction.
          c. F—A small pupil secondary to constrictor spasm is the rule.
          d. T—Adhesions form between the iris and lens.
          e. T—Occurs if the adhesions occlude the pupil causing the iris to bow forward.

A.4.20 a. T
          b. F—Uveitis is by definition an inflammation of the uvea, in this case the choroid.
          c. T
          d. F
          e. F

A.4.21 a. T
          b. T—By a number of mechanisms.
          c. F
          d. T—Often found in Still's disease.
          e. F—Although the reverse is true.

A.4.22 a. T
          b. T—Due to cells and debris in the vitreous.
          c. F
          d. F
          e. F

Diabetes

Q.4.23 Proliferative retinopathy and treatment:

a. Proliferative retinopathy is common in diabetic children
b. Laser retinal photocoagulation with a CO_2 laser is used in diabetic retinopathy
c. Macula oedema is untreatable in diabetic retinopathy
d. 50% of diabetics with proliferative retinopathy will be blind in 5 years if left untreated
e. Cotton wool spots are signs of acute ischaemia

Q.4.24 Diabetic retinopathy:

a. Is the commonest cause of blindness in young people
b. Is only found in insulin-dependent diabetics
c. Responds to laser treatment
d. Is due to impaired choroidal blood flow
e. Is first seen in the peripheral retina

Q.4.25 New vessels may occur at the following sites in diabetics:

a. The optic disc
b. The conjunctiva
c. The iris
d. The macula
e. The peripheral retina

Q.4.26 In the age-onset type II diabetic:

a. Retinopathy is present in approximately 20% of cases on diagnosis
b. Proliferative retinopathy does not occur
c. Visual loss is usually due to an exudative maculopathy
d. Cataract is more common
e. There is an increased incidence of ischaemic optic neuropathy

For answers see over

Answers

A.4.23 a. F—Proliferative retinopathy is virtually never seen in children.
          b. F—The argon laser is the commonest method of treatment.
          c. F—The results of treatment depend on the amount of ischaemic damage to the fovea rather than the amount of oedema.
          d. T
          e. T—They are due to capillary occlusion in the nerve fibre layer, with interruption of axoplasmic flow.

A.4.24 a. T—It is the commonest cause of registration in this country between the ages of 20 and 65 years.
          b. F—Proliferative retinopathy is more common in insulin-dependent diabetics.
          c. T
          d. F
          e. F—Background retinopathy is often first seen on the temporal side of the macula. Proliferative retinopathy may be seen on the optic disc or in the peripheral retina.

A.4.25 a. T—Indicating severe retinal ischaemia that requires pan retinal photocoagulation.
          b. F
          c. T—This may progress to cause rubeotic glaucoma due to occlusion of the trabecular meshwork by vessels and fibrous tissue.
          d. T—This may be difficult to treat.
          e. T—This is now an indication for pan retinal photocoagulation.

A.4.26 a. T—These patients have usually been diabetic for many years prior to diagnosis.
          b. F
          c. T—This is the commonest cause of retinopathy-related visual loss in these patients.
          d. T—And may mask an underlying retinopathy.
          e. T—Occult diabetes should always be excluded in this condition.

Hypertension

Q.4.27 Hypertensive and other vascular retinopathies:

a. Grade II hypertensive retinopathy is reversible with treatment
b. Branch retinal vein occlusion is more common in hypertensive patients
c. Sickle cell retinopathy is common in Caucasians
d. Retinopathy of prematurity is rare over 32 weeks of gestation
e. Drusen are the same as hard exudates

Q.4.28 The following are features of grade III hypertensive retinopathy:

a. Arteriovenous nipping
b. Flame-shaped haemorrhages
c. Cotton wool spots
d. Papilloedema
e. Hard exudates

Q.4.29 The following statements are correct:

a. Ptosis is an important feature of thyrotoxic eye disease
b. The retinal vessels become more tortuous in senile patients
c. Nipping of the veins is a feature of grade II hypertensive retinopathy
d. Flame-shaped haemorrhages occur in the nerve fibre layer of the retina
e. The visual prognosis in central retinal artery occlusion is better than in central retinal vein occlusion

Q.4.30 The following ocular conditions are more common in hypertensives:

a. Chronic simple glaucoma
b. Central retinal vein occlusion
c. Central retinal artery occlusion
d. Cataract
e. Rhegmatogenous retinal detachment

For answers see over

Answers

A.4.27 a. F—The changes in the vessel walls tend to remain in spite
of treatment. The changes seen in grade III and grade IV
can be reversed by treatment.
  b. T
  c. F—It is more common in black races.
  d. F—Infants weighing less than 2000 g and born before 36
weeks should be examined for this.
  e. F—Drusen are degenerative changes in the pigment epithelium.

A.4.28 a. T—Found also in grade II.
  b. T—Superficial retinal haemorrhages are flame shaped.
  c. T—These are signs of microinfarcts and are swollen axons.
  d. F—This would advance the grading to IV.
  e. T—Often grouped in the nerve fibre layer as a macula star.

A.4.29 a. F—Lid retraction is characteristic.
  b. F—The retinal vessels become narrower and straighter in
old age.
  c. T
  d. T
  e. F—Central retinal artery occlusion usually causes complete
blindness. Some degree of recovery is often seen in
central retinal vein occlusion.

A.4.30 a. T
  b. T
  c. T
  d. F
  e. F

Neuro-ophthalmology

Q.4.31 Disc disorders:

   a. Haemorrhages are sometimes seen on normal discs
   b. A cup disc/ratio of 0.8 is normal
   c. Glaucomatous discs are usually pale as well as cupped
   d. Hypermetropia is a cause of pseudo disc oedema
   e. Chronic simple glaucoma is more common in high myopia

Q.4.32 The following signs aid the diagnosis of early papilloedema:

   a. Pallor of the disc
   b. Loss of spontaneous venous pulsation
   c. Infilling of the optic cup
   d. Haemorrhages on the disc surface
   e. Haemorrhages in the peripheral retina

Q.4.33 Some neuro-ophthalmological signs:

   a. Retrobulbar neuritis causes an afferent pupil defect
   b. Pain on ocular movement is a feature of retrobulbar neuritis
   c. Pituitary adenomata cause homonymous hemianopic defects
   d. Papilloedema is a cause of optic atrophy
   e. Dilated retinal veins are a feature of papilloedema

Q.4.34 Internuclear ophthalmoplegia:

   a. Multiple sclerosis is the commonest cause in the under 40s
   b. Produces an "ataxic" nystagmus
   c. Is due to a lesion of the lateral longitudinal fasciculus
   d. Is characterised by nystagmus of the abducting eye and failure of adduction of the other eye
   e. A vascular cause is usual in the elderly

For answers see over

Answers

A.4.31 a. F—The presence of a haemorrhage should always be investigated as an abnormal finding.

        b. F—A cup/disc ratio greater than 0.6 should give rise to the suspicion of glaucoma.

        c. T

        d. T—The hypermetropic disc may resemble papilloedema.

        e. T

A.4.32 a. F—The disc becomes pinker due to increased capillary pressure.

        b. T

        c. T—Due to axonal swelling.

        d. T

        e. F

A.4.33 a. T—The pupil defect may be the only objective evidence of the disease.

        b. T—This is an important feature of the acute stage.

        c. F—They cause bitemporal field defects.

        d. T—Optic atrophy may follow papilloedema.

        e. T

A.4.34 a. T—Which usually resolves.

        b. T—Older text books use this term.

        c. F—The medial longitudinal fasciculus.

        d. T

        e. T—These often do not resolve completely.

Q.4.35 Ptosis and diplopia:

  a. Ptosis is not a feature of Horner's syndrome
  b. Ptosis is a feature of IVth nerve palsy
  c. Ptosis often occurs in acute angle closure glaucoma
  d. Diplopia is a feature of myasthenia gravis
  e. Diplopia is a feature of pituitary tumours

Q.4.36 Adies pupil:

  a. Is a cause of light/near disassociation
  b. Is the commonest cause of a difference in pupil sizes
  c. Is larger than its fellow in moving from a dark to a light room
  d. Is associated with poor accommodation
  e. Is supersensitive to weak solutions of pilocarpine

Q.4.37 The following are important causes of optic atrophy:

  a. Glaucoma
  b. Retinal detachment
  c. Raised intracranial pressure
  d. Chlorpromazine toxicity
  e. Choroidal melanoma

Q.4.38 In myasthenia gravis:

  a. The eyes alone may be involved
  b. Intermittent vertical squints occur
  c. Ptosis is often the only ocular sign
  d. Symptoms may be relieved by the use of neostigmine
  e. This condition is a cause of cataract

Q.4.39 Optic neuritis:

  a. Is a common presenting feature of demyelinating disease
  b. Is associated with constriction of the visual fields
  c. Pallor of the disc is delayed for several weeks
  d. Is usually associated with proptosis
  e. Usually results in permanent blindness on the affected side

For answers see over

Answers

A.4.35 a. F—Slight ptosis is characteristic.
b. F—The IVth cranial nerve has no action on the upper lid.
c. T
d. T—Diplopia becomes worse as the day goes on or as the patient tires.
e. T—IIIrd, IVth or VIth cranial nerve palsies may occur as the tumour expands.

A.4.36 a. F—It is a tonic pupil.
b. F—Essential anisocoria affects 20% of the population.
c. T—It is slow to constrict in light.
d. T—The ciliary ganglion is thought to be affected.
e. T—A case of denervation hypersensitivity.

A.4.37 a. T—The optic atrophy is associated with cupping of the disc.
b. F
c. T—Optic atrophy may follow papilloedema.
d. F—Chlorpromazine can cause cataract in large doses.
e. F

A.4.38 a. T—Ocular myasthenia.
b. T—Often only present when the patient is tired.
c. T—And should be excluded in an isolated case of ptosis.
d. T—This drug is the mainstay of treatment in systemic myasthenia.
e. F—The similar sounding myotonia causes cataract.

A.4.39 a. T—About 30% of patients in the 20–45 years age group subsequently develop demyelinating disease.
b. F—It is associated with paracentral defects in the visual field.
c. T
d. F
e. F—90% of patients recover normal visual acuity after the first attack.

Q.4.40 Visual field defects:

a. Pituitary adenomata typically cause homonymous hemianopias
b. Craniopharyngiomata cause bitemporal hemianopia with the denser scotoma inferiorly
c. Toxic amblyopia causes a centrocaecal scotoma
d. Optic radiation lesions cause homonymous hemianopia with macula sparing
e. Temporal lobe lesions cause an upper quadrantanopia on the side opposite to the lesion

Paediatric Opthalmology

Q.4.41 A strawberry naevus:

a. Usually requires surgery
b. Does not directly invade the globe
c. May cause amblyopia
d. Can be treated with steroid injections
e. Will not grow following birth

Q.4.42 The eyes of a newborn normal fullterm baby:

a. Have an axial length of 24 mm
b. Have pupils which should react to light
c. Have an iris with a slate grey colour
d. Are myopic
e. Are fully coordinated in their movements

Q.4.43 The visual acuity of an infant:

a. Can be measured by the Stycar test
b. Can be measured using reversed Snellen type
c. Is usually less than 6/24
d. Is dependent on cone rather than rod function
e. Can be measured by preferential looking

For answers see over

Answers

A.4.40 a. F—Bitemporal hemianopias, superior fields have denser scotoma.
  b. T—By compression of the posterior chiasmal fibres.
  c. T
  d. F—Occipital lesions cause true macula sparing defects.
  e. T—Due to the pathway of the optic radiations.

A.4.41 a. F—Many resolve spontaneously by the age of 5 years.
  b. T
  c. T—Occurs if the eyelids are closed by the tumour.
  d. T
  e. F—Their initial rapid rate of growth soon after birth slows and is followed by involution.

A.4.42 a. F—This is the adult axial length.
  b. T
  c. T—Due to absence of stromal pigmentation.
  d. F—Slightly hypermetropic.
  e. F—Poor coordination is usual for the first 2 or 3 months.

A.4.43 a. F—But a 3-year-old can sometimes do the Stycar test.
  b. F—Reverse Snellen type is designed to be read through a mirror.
  c. F—When recordable it is usually 6/9 or even better.
  d. T
  e. T—This psychophysical test can be carried out on babies.

Q.4.44 **The following are causes of congenital or developmental cataract:**

a. Galactosaemia
b. Hypocalcaemia
c. Rubella
d. Lowe's syndrome
e. X-ray examination of the mother during pregnancy

Q.4.45 **The following are a cause of leucocoria (white pupil):**

a. Congenital cataract
b. Congenital glaucoma
c. Retinoblastoma
d. Retinopathy of prematurity
e. Congenital convergent squint

Q.4.46 **Retrolental fibroplasia (retinopathy of prematurity):**

a. Was a common cause of infantile blindness in the 1950s
b. Is known to be associated with oxygen therapy
c. Is a type of congenital cataract
d. Is due to rubella infection
e. Is a complication of rheumatoid arthritis

Q.4.47 **Epiphora in an infant may be an important sign of:**

a. Corneal foreign body
b. Buphthalmos
c. The Riley–Day syndrome
d. Blocked nasolacrimal ducts
e. Dominant congenital cataracts

Q.4.48 **The following are common causes of unilateral visual loss in childhood:**

a. Still's disease
b. Anisometropia
c. Amblyopia of disuse
d. Keratoconus
e. Myopia

For answers see over

Answers

A.4.44 a. T—A cause of reversible cataract in infancy
      b. T
      c. T—If acquired by the mother in the first trimester
      d. T—Oculocerebrorenal syndrome.
      e. T

A.4.45 a. T
      b. F
      c. T
      d. T
      e. F

A.4.46 a. T
      b. T—Tends to affect infants who weigh less than 1300 g at birth and who have been exposed to high oxygen concentrations.
      c. F—The lens is usually not involved.
      d. F
      e. F

A.4.47 a. T—And may be the only clue to its presence.
      b. T—Congenital glaucoma causes splits in the layers of the cornea as it enlarges and watering of the eye.
      c. F—This is familial dysautonomia with absent tearing and reduced corneal sensation.
      d. T—As in the adult.
      e. F

A.4.48 a. F—This is a rare cause of unilateral visual loss.
      b. T—Anisometropia tends to lead to amblyopia of disuse.
      c. T—This is a very common cause of unilateral impairment of vision at any age.
      d. F—Keratoconus is usually seen in the early teens.
      e. T

Q.4.49 **In gonococcal ophthalmia neonatorum:**
  a. Symptoms usually appear after the first week of life
  b. Treatment with chloramphenicol is advised
  c. Corneal ulceration is unlikely
  d. Spontaneous resolution is the rule
  e. Maternal infection is rare

Inherited Eye Disease

Q.4.50 **The following show autosomal dominant inheritance:**
  a. Down's syndrome
  b. Colour blindness
  c. Neurofibromatosis
  d. Congenital glaucoma
  e. Ocular albinism

Q.4.51 **In X-linked ocular albinism:**
  a. Only males have reduced vision
  b. Iris transillumination can be elicited
  c. Carrier females may show fundal abnormalities
  d. A sensory congenital type nystagmus occurs
  e. Males can pass on the condition to their sons

Q.4.52 **The following show autosomal recessive inheritance:**
  a. Retinitis pigmentosa
  b. Retinoblastoma
  c. Marfan's syndrome
  d. Refsum's syndrome
  e. Abetalipoproteinaemia

For answers see over

Answers

A.4.49 a. F—Usually within the first 5 days.
  b. F—Frequent application of penicillin or erythromycin drops is advised.
  c. F—The gonococcus can invade healthy corneal epithelium.
  d. F—Corneal scarring and/or perforation will occur if no treatment is given.
  e. F—The parents should be screened for all venereal diseases.

A.4.50 a. F—Associated with chromosomal dysgenesis usually trisomy 21.
  b. F—Usually sex-linked recessive.
  c. T
  d. T
  e. F—Complete albinism inherited as autosomal recessive, ocular albinism as sex-linked recessive.

A.4.51 a. T—Only males have the full syndrome.
  b. T—In both affected males and carrier females.
  c. T—Areas of hypo- and hyperpigmentation may be present.
  d. T—Due to foveal hypoplasia.
  e. F—All sons of affected males will be normal. (Unless the mother is a carrier female!)

A.4.52 a. T—The inheritance may be autosomal dominant, recessive or X-linked.
  b. F—Cases are autosomal dominant or sporadic.
  c. F—Autosomal dominant with variable penetrance.
  d. T—A phytanic acid alpha-hydroxylase deficiency.
  e. T—(d) and (e) are treatable causes of a retinitis pigmentosa-type retinal dystrophy.

Drugs and the Eye

Q.4.53 **The following drugs have antiviral properties:**

a. Proxymetacaine
b. Acetazolamide
c. Acyclovir
d. Idoxuridine
e. Timolol

Q.4.54 **The following have been associated with the use of topical steroids:**

a. Cataract formation
b. Raised intraocular pressure
c. Retinal detachment
d. Herpes simplex keratitis
e. Macular degeneration

Q.4.55 **The following are meiotic agents:**

a. Cocaine
b. Pilocarpine
c. Phospholine iodide
d. Cyclopentolate
e. Timolol

Q.4.56 **The following drugs are known to cause macular degeneration:**

a. Amiodarone
b. Ethambutol
c. Thioridazine
d. Chloroquine
e. Practolol

For answers see over

Answers

A.4.53 a. F—A local anaesthetic.
        b. F—A carbonic anhydrase inhibitor.
        c. T
        d. T
        e. F—A beta blocker.

A.4.54 a. T—But only with the use of large doses.
        b. T—One drop may be enough in susceptible individuals.
        c. F
        d. T—This may cause disastrous effects.
        e. F

A.4.55 a. F
        b. T—This is a cholinergic alkaloid.
        c. T—This is a cholinesterase inhibitor.
        d. F—A mydriatic and cycloplegic agent.
        e. F—A beta blocker.

A.4.56 a. F—Corneal deposition of the drug is seen with the slit lamp.
        b. F—This causes a toxic amblyopia due to optic neuropathy.
        c. T—The only phenothiazine on the market which does.
        d. T—The classical "bull's eye" maculopathy.
        e. F—Causes cicatricial changes in the conjunctiva.

Eye Disease in the Elderly

Q.4.57   Macular degeneration:
   a. Reduces distance vision more than reading vision
   b. Produces reduced peripheral visual fields
   c. Results in loss of colour discrimination
   d. Is treatable with the argon laser in some circumstances
   e. Is associated with colloid body deposition within the pigment epithelium

Q.4.58   The following conditions are more common in the elderly:
   a. Macula holes
   b. Basal cell carcinoma
   c. Ectropion
   d. Chronic simple glaucoma
   e. Dry eye

Q.4.59   Arcus senilis:
   a. Is associated with hyperlipidaemia in the elderly
   b. Is more common in glaucoma
   c. Extends to the limbus
   d. Is a contraindication to cataract extraction
   e. Is a corneal infiltrate

Q.4.60   Patients with macular degeneration:
   a. Should be warned that they will go blind if they live long enough
   b. Cannot be helped by magnifying aids
   c. May lose vision suddenly
   d. Read better in dim light
   e. Can still drive if their vision is 6/18 in each eye

For answers see over

Answers

A.4.57 a. F—Tends to affect the reading vision.
        b. F—Affects central field.
        c. T
        d. T—In cases where choroidal new vessels threaten the foveal region.
        e. T—Colloid bodies may be seen in the macula region some years before the vision becomes impaired.

A.4.58 a. T
        b. T
        c. T
        d. T—The incidence rises progressively over the age of 45 years.
        e. T

A.4.59 a. F—A juvenile arcus however, is associated with hyperlipidaemia.
        b. F
        c. F—There is usually a clear marginal zone.
        d. F
        e. T—It is an annular stromal infiltrate with lipid material.

A.4.60 a. F—Quite the opposite; the progress is very variable and navigational vision is retained.
        b. F—Many aids are available ranging from a simple magnifying glass to closed-circuit television.
        c. T—Due to sudden macula haemorrhage from a disciform lesion.
        d. F—The opposite is true.
        e. F—This would fall below the legal driving limit.

Questions

Q.4.61 Cranial arteritis:

a. Often presents with loss of vision in one eye
b. Is rare over the age of 60 years
c. Should be treated with low doses of steroids initially
d. Is a cause of diplopia
e. Is a cause of stroke

Q.4.62 A right homonymous hemianopia from a stroke:

a. Is often not noticed by the patient
b. Can cause reading difficulties with 6/6 vision in each eye
c. Is often described as "poor vision in my right eye"
d. Is never associated with visual agnosia
e. Usually recovers fully

Q.4.63 In the management of chronic simple glaucoma in the elderly:

a. Acetazolamide can cause mental confusion
b. Pilocarpine is contraindicated
c. Timolol can cause cardiac failure
d. Macular degeneration contradindicates treatment
e. Siblings are rarely affected

Q.4.64 Diabetes in the elderly may cause:

a. An ischaemic optic neuropathy
b. A VIth nerve palsy
c. Macular oedema
d. A dislocated lens
e. Vitreous haemorrhage

Q.4.65 The following conditions are common in the elderly:

a. Buphthalmos
b. Entropion
c. Angioid striae
d. Small pupils
e. Arcus juvenalis

For answers see over

Answers

A.4.61
  a. T—May present with central retinal artery occlusion.
  b. F—It is rare under the age of 60 years.
  c. F—High doses over 100 mg prednisolone are advised initially in a confirmed case.
  d. T
  e. T

A.4.62
  a. T—It produces a "negative" scotoma.
  b. T—Scanning into the lost visual field renders reading difficult.
  c. T—A trap for the unwary.
  d. F—An inability to recognise familiar objects may accompany a right homonymous hemianopia.
  e. F—Although some recovery may occur, patients are usually left with the handicap and should not drive.

A.4.63
  a. T—Carbonic anhydrase inhibitors are "metabolic poisons".
  b. F—The poor accommodational reserve and small pupils found in the elderly ease tolerance.
  c. T—By systemic absorption and lowering of the cardiac output.
  d. F—The remaining peripheral field may otherwise be extinguished by the glaucoma.
  e. F—Siblings have a 10%–20% chance of having glaucoma.

A.4.64
  a. T—Diabetes should be excluded when this occurs.
  b. T—Diabetes should be excluded when this occurs.
  c. T—Diabetic maculopathy.
  d. F
  e. T—From proliferative retinopathy.

A.4.65
  a. F—Buphthalmos is caused by congenital glaucoma.
  b. T
  c. F—This is a rare appearance seen typically in association with pseudo-xanthoma elasticum of the skin.
  d. T—The pupils become smaller with age.
  e. F—This is a lipid infiltrate of the peripheral cornea seen in young patients.

Q.4.66 In the elderly:
   a. Binocular vision is usually lost
   b. Prismatic spectacles are contraindicated
   c. Local anaesthesia is poorly tolerated
   d. Intraocular lens insertion is the commonest optical correction for aphakia
   e. Loss of vision from trauma is commoner than in young adults

Q.4.67 Senile macula degeneration:
   a. Is associated with colloid bodies
   b. Causes tunnel vision
   c. Occurs in 1% of patients over 70 years
   d. Shows a slow response to local steroids
   e. Is the commonest cause of blindness in the over 60s

Q.4.68 Temporal arteritis:
   a. Is best diagnosed by biopsy of the temporal artery
   b. Often presents with pain around the jaw
   c. Is characterised by painful pulsating temporal arteries
   d. Is most common in middle age
   e. Requires immediate treatment with steroids to prevent blindness

For answers see over

Answers

A.4.66 a. F
   b. F—They may be the best way of aiding a muscle balance problem.
   c. F—On the whole it is well tolerated.
   d. T
   e. F—The young adult male and children are most at risk.

A.4.67 a. T
   b. F—Causes a central scotoma.
   c. F—Occurs in about 8% of the 65–75 years age group.
   d. F—So far no proven response to medical treatment.
   e. T—In the Western world.

A.4.68 a. T—This is the surest way to reach a firm diagnosis but a repeat biopsy may be needed if the first is negative.
   b. T
   c. F—The arteries may be painful but do not pulsate.
   d. F—More common over the age of 70 years.
   e. T—Especially if there are visual symptoms.

5. *Blindness*

Q.5.1   **The following are benefits from blind registration in the UK:**

a. Free TV licence
b. Disabled badge for sighted relative's car
c. Additional income tax relief
d. A talking book
e. A free radio

Q.5.2   **Other facts:**

a. A patient is classified as blind if the vision is worse than "hand movements"
b. Telescopic lenses are useful if the vision is not worse than 6/12
c. The mean survival time following registration as blind from glaucoma is 18 months
d. The incidence of blindness is about 5% of the population in the Western world
e. No blind pension is available in the UK at present

Q.5.3   **Patients can be registered as partially sighted if their vision is 6/6 in each eye and:**

a. They have a homonymous hemianopia
b. They have an altitudinal defect in one eye
c. They have red/green colour blindness
d. They have constricted visual fields from glaucoma
e. They have aphakic glasses

Q.5.4   **More about classification of visual handicap:**

a. Patients can be registered partially sighted if they lose vision in one eye
b. A patient with a visual acuity of 6/24 can be registered as partially sighted in the UK.
c. Vitamin A deficiency causes colour blindness
d. Most patients on the blind register can read Braille
e. One-eyed patients cannot acquire a Heavy Goods Vehicle licence

For answers see over

Answers

A.5.1 a. F—A small decrease only is allowed.
      b. T
      c. T
      d. T
      e. T—From the local social services.

A.5.2 a. F—Blind registration is considered if the vision in both eyes is worse than 6/60 or sometimes better if there is severe impairment of the visual field.
      b. F—The use of telescopic lenses is more dependent on the age and reading desires of the patient and they may be useful when the vision is down to 6/60.
      c. F—It is 10 years.
      d. F—The incidence is less than 1%.
      e. F

A.5.3 a. T—And of course they should be advised against driving.
      b. F—The eye with the full field precludes registration.
      c. F
      d. T—Gross field loss may sometimes occur with normal Snellen acuity.
      e. F

A.5.4 a. F—A one-eyed person need not suffer serious employment difficulty.
      b. T
      c. F—Vitamin A deficiency causes night blindness.
      d. F—Most elderly patients find Braille difficult to learn.
      e. T

GPSR Compliance

*The European Union's (EU) General Product Safety Regulation (GPSR)
is a set of rules that requires consumer products to be safe and our
obligations to ensure this.*

*If you have any concerns about our products, you can contact us on
ProductSafety@springernature.com*

In case Publisher is established outside the EU, the EU authorized
representative is:

Springer Nature Customer Service Center GmbH
Europaplatz 3
69115 Heidelberg, Germany

Batch number: 09635029

Printed by Printforce, the Netherlands